STO

Is Surgery Necessary?

Is Surgery Necessary?

Siegfried J. Kra, M.D., F.A.C.P.

Robert S. Boltax, M.D., F.A.C.S.

MACMILLAN PUBLISHING CO., INC.

NEW YORK

Copyright © 1981 by Siegfried J. Kra
and Robert S. Boltax

Macmillan Publishing Co., Inc.
866 Third Avenue, New York, N.Y. 10022
Collier Macmillan Canada, Ltd.

Library of Congress Cataloging in Publication Data

Kra, Siegfried J
    Is surgery necessary?

    1. Surgery—Popular works.   2. Surgery,
Unnecessary.   3. Patient education.   I. Boltax,
Robert S., joint author.   II. Title. [DNLM:
1. Referral and consultation.   2. Surgery.
WO 64 K89i]
RD31.3.K7   617   80-26996
ISBN 0-02-566560-X

10 9 8 7 6 5 4 3 2 1

Printed in the United States of America

To our patients and teachers
who inspired us to write this book

"Opinion is the main thing which does good or harm in the world. It is our false opinion of things which ruin us."

Marcus Aurelius

Contents

Acknowledgments

THIS BOOK IS MADE POSSIBLE through the excellent advice and review of manuscripts by the following distinguished, world-renowned physicians: Dr. Samuel Thier, David Paige Smith Professor and chairman of Department of Internal Medicine, Yale School of Medicine; Dr. Lawrence Cohen, professor of medicine, Department of Cardiology, Yale School of Medicine; Dr. Philip Felig, C H N Long Professor of Medicine, director of General Clinical Research Center, and vice chairman of Department of Medicine, Yale School of Medicine; Dr. Ira Goldenberg, clinical professor of surgery, Yale School of Medicine; Dr. Donald Coustan, assistant professor of obstetrics and gynecology, Yale School of Medicine; Dr. Ronald Cwik, clinical instructor of obstetrics and gynecology, Yale School of Medicine; Dr. Bernard Lytton, professor of urology, Department of Urology, Yale School of Medicine; Dr. Peter Demir, clinical instructor of urology, Yale School of Medicine; Dr. Stephen Stein, assistant clinical professor of surgery, Yale School of Medicine; Dr. Robert Margolis, assistant professor of

[xi]

orthopedic surgery, Yale School of Medicine; Dr. Gustave
Sirot, associate clinical professor of dermatology, Yale School
of Medicine; Dr. Harold Stern, associate clinical professor of
cardiothoracic surgery, Yale School of Medicine; Dr. Allan
Toole, assistant clinical professor of cardiothoracic surgery,
Yale School of Medicine; Dr. Howard Spiro, professor of
medicine, Department of Gastroenterology, Yale School of
Medicine; Dr. Robert Aaronson, assistant clinical professor of
medicine, Department of Gastroenterology, Yale School of
Medicine; Dr. Isaac Goodrich; Dr. Boris Rifkin, assistant clinical
professor of psychiatry, Yale School of Medicine; Dr. Theo-
dore Zanker, assistant clinical professor of psychiatry, Yale
School of Medicine; Dr. Emily Fine, resident in obstetrics and
gynecology, Yale School of Medicine; Dr. Keat-Jin Lee, M.D.,
clinical instructor of otolaryngology, Yale School of Medicine;
Dr. Joseph Dineen, chief of surgery, Griffin Hospital, assistant
clinical professor of cardiothoracic surgery, Yale School of
Medicine; Dr. Francis J. Scarpa, clinical instructor of surgery,
Yale School of Medicine; the staff of the Hospital of St.
Raphael; special thanks to Renee Kra for her excellent advice
on editing and Marcelle Boltax for her endless encouragement;
thanks also to Ferenc A. Gyorgyey, Historical Librarian, Yale
Historical Library Medical Library, and to the hundreds of
practicing physicians who gave their second opinions.*

SECOND OPINION

Thousands of Americans face surgery each year, often with fear
and with doubts about whether the right step is being taken.
Surgery is often necessary. However, it may not always be the only
way to treat a particular health problem.

How can we know for sure?

A major consumer information campaign by the U.S. Department
of Health, Education, and Welfare is underway to encourage all citi-

*We also gratefully acknowledge the invaluable help of Madelyn Munson,
who typed this manuscript.

zens, on a voluntary basis, to seek a second professional opinion before undergoing non-emergency surgery.

The reassurance of a second opinion from another doctor can build confidence and alleviate fears for a patient by supplying enough information to make a choice about whether or not to have non-emergency surgery. A second opinion better enables people to weigh the benefits and risks of having an operation against the benefits and risks of not having one and to consider possible alternatives to surgery.

The practice of medicine is not an exact science. Physicians do not always agree. This does not reflect on their competency or their concern to do what is best for their patients. It simply means that there can be differences of opinion about the best ways to treat a specific medical condition.

Second opinions are a long and honored practice in the medical profession. Many physicians seek a second opinion for their patients—and for themselves—prior to ordering or undergoing surgery.

When non-emergency surgery is recommended, a patient should learn, through a second opinion, the benefits, risks, and alternatives to the recommended surgery.

HEW suggests four ways to locate a specialist to give a second opinion*:

- Ask your doctor to refer you to another doctor who is a specialist in the specific medical condition.
- Call the HEW toll-free number, 800-325-6400, to locate a specialist in your community.
- If eligible for Medicaid, contact your local welfare office to see if your state will pay for a second surgical opinion.
- If covered by Medicare, call your local Social Security office.

Additional information can be obtained by writing Surgery, Washington, D.C. 20201.

*From a HEW news item sent to physicians, hospitals, and paramedical personnel. Date 1978

Introduction

ONE IN TEN AMERICANS will undergo some surgical procedure in the coming year. Over twenty million operations will be performed at a cost of billions of dollars, at annual increases of 5 percent per year. Some public health authorities claim that the continued increase of surgery is not justified and reflects over-zealous surgeons eager to practice their skill.

The U.S. Department of Health and Human Services officially promotes the idea of seeking a second opinion before under-going nonemergency surgery. Insurance carriers applaud the idea, as this will cut down on claims, while the public is left in the middle, confused and now questioning its traditional faith in physicians.

Most surgical operations performed today are warranted. Each hospital has a watchdog committee that reviews all the pathological specimens removed at surgery. It is unlikely that today, in our sophisticated medical society, repeated unwar-ranted surgery occurs. This book is not written to defend the medical profession, but to enlighten the patient so he can make a proper choice and understand if surgery is necessary.

Two viewpoints are presented when indicated: the surgeon's and the internist's. This is essential, as surgeons may tend to agree with one another, as, for example, when a gall bladder should be removed.

When the patient is confronted with a surgical problem and then seeks a second opinion, he is relieved when the second opinion affirms the first, but becomes chagrined and confused when the second opinion differs from the first. Where shall he go then? To a third opinion? And then to whom does he listen?

A recent example comes to mind of a patient in our community who was advised by the medical center to have a surgical procedure performed. Taking advantage of the new insurance carriers' law, the patient went to another renowned surgical center in the West and was advised not to have the surgical procedure. In effect, the patient's dilemma was compounded by having a third astute opinion, which agreed with the first. The husband of the patient was still dissatisfied and went to a fourth medical center, which agreed with the second opinion, and on it went.

An educated and informed patient is able to make better decisions and pose succinct, pertinent questions to his doctor with the hope of receiving honest, direct, thoughtful answers.

The material contained in this text arises from years of experience and from obtaining the consensus of opinions from some of the top surgeons in the United States and abroad. We cannot cover every surgical procedure, but plan to limit ourselves to the most controversial surgical operations performed. For example, when the diagnosis for acute appendicitis is firmly made, a second opinion is not warranted, as surgery must be done quickly, efficiently, and time should not be spent seeking a second opinion at three o'clock in the morning. On the other hand, with conditions that have been present for a lengthy period of time, such as stones in the gallbladder, fibroid tumor, hernias, and numerous other conditions that we are going to discuss, a second opinion may be warranted.

Is Surgery Necessary?

1: The Gold Bladder (Gallbladder)

We have titled this chapter The Gold Bladder, since one billion dollars per year are spent for surgery on this structure. Most of the surgery is performed on patients between the ages of forty and sixty-five, with an average hospital stay of ten days, and, undoubtedly, gallbladder surgery is increasing as the incidence of stone formation rises. The cause of this increase will become evident to the reader as we briefly outline what the gallbladder is, its function, how stones form, and why they cause the illness in the first place.

Function of the Gallbladder

The gallbladder is a small sac with a capacity of approximately 1½ ounces. The liver produces nearly 1 liter of bile per day and most of this is reabsorbed by the wall of the gallbladder. It is located on the right side of the abdomen, under the liver, protruding downward, and comes into intimate contact with the stomach, pancreas, and other surrounding organs.

The gallbladder functions as a storage house for the bile that is secreted by the liver. It is the bile that allows us to digest our food, especially fats. The bile looks very similar to urine and contains many chemical substances, such as bile pigment, cholesterol, fats, soaps, fatty acids, lecithin, proteins, and numerous others. The bile that is found in the gallbladder is a different color than is excreted from the liver. It is dark—gold-brown to almost pitch black in color, depending on the concentration of cholesterol pigment and bile salts. The gallbladder replenishes its supply of bile usually during fasting, overnight, between meals, and after the stomach has emptied itself. Normally, during the periods between eating, the entire flow of bile from the liver is carried into the gallbladder. Some of it also goes into the small intestine. By means of valves, the bile flows from the gallbladder into the intestines. Included in the bile contents are water, sodium, chloride, bicarbonate, and calcium.

When the gallbladder becomes diseased either by an inflammation of its walls or when filled with stones, the flow of bile and digestion are impaired. We suffer from indigestion and/or pain. If the gallbladder is inflamed, we speak of cholecystitis. The condition of stones in the gallbladder is called cholelithiasis.

Gallstones and How They Form

Gallstones occur in two main types, depending on their basic composition. Both types of stones are not dissolved in water or in bile. The first, called cholesterol stones, consists of a mixture of phospholipids and bile acids (bile acids are detergents derived from the breakdown of cholesterol). These stones are usually single but may be many in number. They are lightweight, white, with a radiant surface, glittering with crystals of cholesterol, varying in size from a pea to an apple. Seen on the operating table, they look like a bean sack filled with collected terrestrial stones. They are hard in consistency and would be an effective weapon if used in a slingshot.

The second major type of stone is composed mostly of calcium combined with bilirubin and other pigments which result from the breakdown of hemoglobin. In some blood disorders red blood cells are destroyed continuously, as in congenital hemolytic anemias, and stone formation is a common accompaniment of the illness. They contain very little cholesterol and are referred to as pigment stones. Pure pigment stones are small and dark in color.

A third group, sometimes called mixed stones, contains both pigment and cholesterol. A mixed stone may occur singly, occupying the entire sac, or be multiple in number. When we examine the mixed stone lying on the table, it will have many facets corresponding to its proximity to the other stones. Its cut surface is adorned with concentric plates, as the under-surface of a mushroom or the gills of a clam. The pathologist refers to these as *lamella formations.*

Stone formation represents an intriguing complicated mishap in the metabolic events of the body. They are a by-product of abnormal pathways. Much controversy exists as to why and how they form, and they are under constant scrutiny by biochemists and physiologists.

The following general steps lead to stone formation: First, the gallbladder becomes overstuffed with bile that is too rich and concentrated—called *super-saturated*—with cholesterol, pigments, and other chemicals. These substances then arrange themselves into a nidus or nucleus and then attract more and more crystals on their initial surface until they are full grown and matured. This genesis of the stone is not completed on the sixth day—it is not really known how long stone formation takes.

Certain favorable settings are necessary for stones to begin their growth. A continued flow of bile occurs between the liver, intestines, and gallbladder: materials added and removed from the bile, stimulated by chemical reactions or simply by a fatty meal. The gallbladder must contract vigorously to empty itself when stimulated. When it becomes sluggish and lazy, as during pregnancy, in illnesses such as diabetes, and with some gastrointestinal diseases, the bile stagnates and the setting is now ripe for stones to form.

Excessive ingestion of rich foods containing cholesterol substances overload the bile with this fat, and stones form. Obese females are expert stone makers, especially of the cholesterol variety. Their gallbladders become repositories for cholesterol and Fort Knoxes for surgeons.

In our rich fat-laden nation cholesterol stones appear during the mature years—the coronary years. In northern Europe and North and South America, cholesterol stones predominate, while pigment stones tend to be more prevalent in the Orient. Over the past decade a shift has been occurring in Japan, where pigment stones are becoming less and cholesterol stones more frequent. Pigment stones tend to occur in conditions in which the life span of the red blood cell is decreased, as occurs in certain hereditary blood illnesses; likewise, it appears that alcoholics and those with cirrhosis have more pigment stones. Pigment stones are rare among American Indians, but they have a very high incidence of cholesterol stones. Other ethnic groups, such as the Masai of Africa, rarely have stones.

The increase in incidence of stones among females has been documented time and time again. It begins at the age of puberty and diminishes after the menopause. It is not clear why women have an increased incidence of stones as compared to men, except that women do have more amounts of total bile acids than men, and the more the bile acid, the more cholesterol there is in the gallbladder.

Sluggishness of the gallbladder has been observed in women during the mid-phase of their menstrual cycle, and women definitely empty their gallbladders much more slowly than men. Such sluggish emptying contributes to increased stone formation.

Obese females and people whose diets contain large amounts of cholesterol are predisposed to form cholesterol stones.

The use of oral contraceptives and estrogens seems to increase the incidence of gall stones. The Food and Drug Administration now requires that a warning of increased risk of gallbladder disease be included in the patient's package insert distributed with all contraceptives.

High cholesterol is sometimes treated with a medication called clofibrate or Atromid-S. Although this drug prevents cholesterol formation, it is associated with more cholesterol secretion and formation of stones. Other substances for the treatment of high cholesterol have now been implicated in the formation of stones in the gallbladder.

Symptoms of Gallbladder Disease

Doctors have long described the picture of the patient with cholelithiasis by the eponym: Fat, Forty, Flatulent, and Female. Gallbladder disease can occur in the teen-ager or make its first appearance at the age of eighty as an acute attack.

Pain may occur in the abdomen in an intermittent mild colicky fashion, or as a sudden terrifying sensation of pain in the stomach accompanied with vomiting. The patient may have suffered for years with nagging complaints of "I am so bloated, so full, so gassy, so distended, especially after a greasy meal." After having a diet laden with creams, a general nonspecific discomfort with pain in the right upper quadrant of the abdomen may follow. Sometimes the only symptom of a diseased gallbladder or stone may be heartburn after eating or recurrent episodes of nausea and vomiting.

During an acute attack the patient might look pale and perspiring, with shaking chills, wide-eyed, fearful, and thrashing about, unable to find a comfortable position. The patient with severe pain will visit the emergency room and will have studies performed to rule out a heart attack, as these two illnesses sometimes are confused or appear together.

In even more severe cases, the patient may present with jaundice, as evidenced by a slight yellow tinge in the eyes and skin. This occurs when one of the small stones passes the outlet of the gallbladder, called the *cystic duct,* and then floats into the main duct, called the *common bile duct.* Bacteria may then enter and cause an infection that spreads to the liver and its canals, termed *cholangitis,* a dreaded complication for the patient and a surgeon's nightmare which can lead to possible surgical emergency and even death. Another dire complication of the diseased gallbladder is an inflamed pancreas, called *pancreatitis,* which requires very specialized treatment.

The Diagnosis of Gallbladder Disease

The physician will readily diagnose a diseased gallbladder from the history and physical examination if the classical symptoms described are present. Atypical symptoms sometimes occur, as chest pain rather than pain in the stomach. Rarely, pain in the right shoulder has been described.

GALLBLADDER X-RAY EXAMINATION

Appropriate laboratory tests and X-ray examinations will confirm the diagnosis. The routine X-ray examination is called a *gallbladder series.* Provided that the patient is not nauseated and vomiting, he is given pills, called Telepaque, that have an iodine base. They are taken the night before the examination and are absorbed into the bloodstream from the intestines. After being removed by cells of the liver, the dye is excreted into the bile and passed into the gallbladder. X rays taken the following morning will disclose either stones or the gallbladder will not be visualized. If the gallbladder is normal, the normal empty sac will be seen. If the gallbladder is not visualized, it may be abnormal, secondary to infection, or so diseased that it cannot concentrate the material because of the presence of stones. A stone lodged at the outlet of the gallbladder may prevent the dye material from entering. If the patient is too ill to swallow the pills, the dye is injected into the vein and the biliary tree is observed. Concomitantly with the gallbladder X ray, the physician may order an X ray of the stomach, called a gastrointestinal series, as some of the symptoms of gallbladder disease may also be similar to symptoms of stomach disorders. Laboratory tests also include liver and pancreas studies.

Recently a new test has been added to the armamentarium for diagnosing gastrointestinal diseases—the *ultrasonic* examination. Sound waves are passed into the abdomen, reflected back, and an image is obtained. The sound waves are not X rays. They have proven to be remarkably accurate for the evaluation of areas of the abdomen and for the gallbladder. The major handicap of the examination is that it may be difficult to visualize a stone if the intestine is distended with a lot of gas. Ultrasonic examination is performed if the gallbladder series is not diagnostic or in the event that the patient cannot take pills as described. Someday ultrasonic examination of the abdomen may entirely replace the conventional gallbladder X rays.

Typical Case Example

Mrs. Robinson swayed her corpulent body uncomfortably in the chair as she described her symptoms to her family physician. She had come to consult her physician because of severe abdominal pain that she had experienced earlier that morning in the upper part of her belly and underneath her rib margin.

"We went to dinner last night," she told the physician. "I ate veal parmesan and drank a glass of wine and had strawberry shortcake for dessert. I woke up at four A.M. with pain and I vomited. I took some Digel and it didn't help."

"Did you ever have this pain before?" the physician asked.

"No," Mrs. Robinson said, "but for the past four months I have felt bloated, especially after eating any fried foods and ice cream. I have been burping a lot and am passing gas."

"Did anybody in your family ever have trouble with their gallbladder?"

"Yes, my mother had stones in her gallbladder, as well as my sister."

Her doctor examined Mrs. Robinson and found this forty-eight-year-old female who was 5 feet 6 inches and weighed 210 pounds to have pain on the right side of the abdomen when he pushed his hand underneath the rib cage. The following day she had a gallbladder X-ray examination, which confirmed the diagnosis of cholelithiasis, and her doctor advised an operation.

Treatment of Cholelithiasis

Once the diagnosis of cholelithiasis, or stones in the gallbladder, has been made, two common avenues of treatment are available: 1) dietary, and 2) surgical.

The surgeons regard disease of the gallbladder primarily as their domain, while the internists look upon the gallbladder as a medical problem. Both are correct, as there is structural abnormality combined with a metabolic derangement which causes the illness in the first place; therefore, surgical and medical treatment go hand in hand in this illness. The surgeon's inclination is to operate, while the medical man, as a rule, is conservative in his approach. However, both will agree in some definite circumstances.

The physician recognizes four groups of patients suffering from gallbladder disease. The first is known to have had several gallbladder attacks and has managed properly with diet, remaining pain free. This first group of patients can remain symptom free for the remainder of their lives. The second group of patients are the ones who have never had an attack before but are seen for the first time in the emergency room, or who have had several attacks and are now considered for surgery. The third group are those who are extremely ill, with long-standing stones in the gallbladder, who arrive with chills, fever, and jaundice, sometimes accompanied by an inflammation of the pancreas. The fourth group, which is the most controversial, comprises those patients with silent stones. The enormous increase of routine X-ray examinations has uncovered thousands of symptom-free patients with stones in their gallbladders.

The patient who arrives acutely ill, with jaundice and accompanying pancreatitis, requires urgent and proper treatment to regain optimal condition. A second opinion will only delay the proper care of these patients, as there is no other alternative but to perform surgery. This situation arises when the stone has traveled out of the gallbladder and into the main duct from the liver to the intestines; the stone obstructs the main duct and prevents the flow of bile. The patient becomes jaundiced and may develop inflammation of the pancreas. As the stone is lodged in the main duct, it prevents a proper flow of bile and the bile backs up into the liver and into the bloodstream, under the skin, which gives the patient a jaundiced appearance. When there is infection accompanying the blockage, the situation is life threatening, especially if there is accompanying sepsis and shock.

A second opinion is warranted in the following illustration. A middle-aged patient is admitted into the hospital because of a severe gallbladder attack. In a few days, with appropriate medical treatment, the patient becomes symptom free. Should this patient have the gallbladder removed?

SURGICAL POINT OF VIEW

The surgeon will contend that a middle-aged patient or a young patient will not be satisfied with spending his entire life on a strict diet and be in constant danger of an attack at a most inconvenient time or place, as on a plane, on a cruise, or visiting the High Lama at Nepal. Furthermore, future complications, such as pancreatitis, may occur. Even though the patient may have no further attacks, he may be constantly uncomfortable—bloating, belching, and feeling full—and these symptoms may not be acceptable. It is always better to operate under ideal circumstances—not as an emergency—well planned in advance.

The complications of gallbladder surgery will depend on how well the patient is before surgery. The young adult who is asymptomatic will rarely have complications, such as infections and a prolonged course in the hospital. The complications will depend on the length of time that the surgeon has to operate, the patient's age (the older the patient the higher the probability of complications), his general physical state prior to surgery (if the patient is jaundiced and infected, his hospitalization will be prolonged in order to adequately treat the infection), and the skill of the surgeon. The complications may consist of 1) postoperative wound infections, which are now readily controlled with a large store of antibiotics and careful wound care, 2) pneumonia and other lung problems, 3) phlebitis and clots to the lung, 4) occasional heart failure, and 5) operative errors—damage to the surrounding organs. All of the above can lead to death.

The mortality rate from surgery in those patients who are relatively symptom free is less than one-tenth of 1 percent. When the patient is acutely ill with fever and jaundice, the mortality rate can swiftly rise to 10 percent. Surgery should be delayed or postponed indefinitely if the patient has severe heart disease, lung disease, or kidney failure. After a heart attack surgery should be delayed for six months to one year, as the mortality is too high during this time, cited as 50 percent in some statistics.

If stones are found on a routine gallbladder series and the patient is asymptomatic, the surgeon will advise an operation if the patient is a young person, especially a young female. A young female who has cholelithiasis should also be operated on electively prior to becoming pregnant. Pregnancy causes relaxation of the smooth muscles, resulting in delay of emptying the gallbladder, and acute attacks can occur during pregnancy. Surgery then may become mandatory, at a significant risk to the fetus and the woman.

A young or middle-aged man with recurrent bouts of acute, painful gallbladder disease should also have surgery. It is better to operate when the patient is pale rather than yellow—the dreaded complications.

If the gallbladder is filled with multiple small stones, the danger of passage of the stones and obstruction is great, and surgery is also recommended, even if only one attack has occurred.

Medical Treatment of Gallbladder Disease

If the patient follows a prescribed complete fat-free diet, he may never again be troubled with gallbladder attacks. A fat-free diet is prescribed because fat stimulates the pancreas to produce hormones which in turn cause the gallbladder to contract. The contracting gallbladder can extrude a small stone, which blocks the outlet from the gallbladder and causes the aforementioned complications.

Sticking to a strict diet is less troublesome than undergoing surgery. If one attack has occurred, there is no way of predicting that another is bound to happen. There is a risk with surgery—granted, it is small, but people have died from the procedure. There is no guarantee that surgery will eliminate the symptoms of belching, bloating, and abdominal distention. After surgery some patients still have the same symptoms, some of which may reflect a psychosomatic syndrome. A small stone may not be detected at surgery in spite of a scrupulous search, and the patient may need to be operated on again.

If another attack does occur, the internist will agree with the surgeon that it is necessary to remove the gallbladder.

There is a new era on the medical horizon in the treatment of cholelithiasis, which, in reality, is primarily a medical illness resulting from a metabolic derangement. Efforts to dissolve stones have been tried for generations, terminating in failure. Treatment has included purgatives, fatty meals, and herbs, all of which usually make the patient worse.

Epidemiological studies have presented evidence that stone formation, or cholelithiasis, is associated with obesity. For example, during wartime decreased caloric intake was associated with a lowered incidence of gallstone formation. A high-caloric diet in our country is synonymous with a high-fat diet; cholesterol absorption is increased and stone formations of the cholesterol variety are augmented. As most stones in the gallbladder contain cholesterol monohydrade and the bile in nearly all individuals is nearly saturated cholesterol, it follows that for cholesterol gallstones to form, the bile must be overwhelmed with cholesterol. The management of gallstones has been directed in the past ten years by the following discoveries: bile acids—called chenodeoxycholic acid—and ursodeoxycholic, when fed by mouth, decrease the amount of cholesterol in the bile and actually dissolve gall stones of the cholesterol variety.

Bile acids are substances secreted from the liver. The administration of bile acids, sometimes called chenic acids for convenience, decreases the amount of cholesterol that accumulates in the bile. The bile ducts become depleted of cholesterol and stones dissolve. Again, only cholesterol gallstones dissolve. Not all cholesterol stones dissolve, as some may be coated with calcium. And, as mentioned before, not all stones are cholesterol in type.

In a study performed by Dr. Alan Hoffman, professor of medicine at the University of California in San Diego, on four thousand patients, no side effects have been seen with the use of this treatment. Treatment, which is still experimental at this time, sometimes requires thirty months before complete dissolution of stones occurs. Chenic acid is now licensed in Europe and South American countries, but, for the time being, is not available in the United States.

Asymptomatic stones in the gallbladder are found in one of ten autopsies. Cholelithiasis is a very common illness of our society, and most internists will not advise surgery until the patient becomes symptomatic.

In the future, patients suffering from chronic stone formation in their gallbladder may have an alternative to surgery. Those who are suffering from recurrent acute attacks will require surgery; however, those patients who have one or two attacks, or none at all, may look forward to having medical treatment of their illness, consisting of strict weight reduction, low-fat diet, and medications of the type of bile acids or chenic acid which will dissolve, at least, cholesterol stones. However, since it takes more than six months to one year for stones to be dissolved, the patient who suffers recurrent attacks and severe discomfort should not have to wait a year to get better. We can only urge these patients to undergo gallbladder surgery.

The controversy of the management of the "silent stone"—asymptomatic stones—found in the gallbladder will soon be settled in part, once chenic acids or like substances are approved for use in the United States.

2: Cardiovascular Surgery

CORONARY ARTERY SURGERY

Heart disease is the number one killer in the United States. It is estimated that each year 1.3 million people sustain a heart attack and 675,000 die from this dreadful illness. In the United States there are four million people suffering with coronary artery disease, all having a history of either a heart attack or angina pectoris.

Coronary artery bypass surgery is currently in fashion as part of the tool kit for the treatment of this malady; cardiac catheterization is the method used to visualize the arteries supplying the heart. Both procedures are a continual source of controversy amongst doctors and of bewilderment to the patient.

Coronary artery disease results when the arteries supplying the heart are clogged with cholesterol, tissue, and other substances. It is a chronic progressive illness beginning in early life and ending with the death of the patient. When the artery becomes critically dammed up, barring any flow of blood and oxygen to the heart, many patients suffer chest pain, called angina; others sustain a heart attack (myocardial infarction); still others die suddenly.

The Anatomy of the Coronary Arteries

Galen, in the year A.D. 130, used the term *coronary* to describe the arteries that supply the heart. Leonardo da Vinci, in the year 1452, sketched the artery vessels in the way we are accustomed to seeing them now. Rudimentary notions of coronary arteries were known during ancient Egyptian times, as described in the Papyrus Papers.

There are two major vessels that arise from the aorta—a left artery and a right artery. Just as there are differences in eye and skin color and in fingerprints, there are also variations in the way the heart is supplied by these arteries. In general terms, the left main artery supplies the front of the heart and the right artery supplies the back of the heart. The left main artery quickly divides from its beginning into a left anterior descending artery and the circumflex coronary artery. It is the left anterior descending branch of the left main artery that supplies the left side of the heart. This branch supplies the wall that separates the right and left side of the heart.

The Symptoms of Coronary Artery Disease

When the coronary arteries become critically narrowed and the heart receives inadequate blood, and, thus, oxygen, the patient may complain of a characteristic pain in his chest. *Angina pectoris*, translated from the Latin, means "pain in the chest," a symptom of a disease process involving the coronary arteries.

Angina consists of periodic attacks of a distinctive pain, usually situated behind the breastbone, radiating to the left side of the chest, down to the inner side of the left arm, and sometimes to other areas, precipitated by effort and relieved by rest or nitroglycerine. The pain may be located behind the middle of the upper third or fourth rib. Sometimes the pain may be felt as soreness, with a choking sensation accompanied by anguish and despair. A sensation of strangling may be felt, of suffocation, oppression, or panic. It may be of a very mild nature that the patient ignores, or it may be severe. Sometimes there is no pain at all, but only a tired or weak feeling.

Characteristically, the patient is seen making a fist, clutching his chest, bending over slightly with shoulders stooped, sometimes perspiring and looking pale. There are numerous variations of the pain, described as burning, sticking pain felt in the arms, the wrists, the jaw, the gums, and the back. The pain may be precipitated by anxiety, cold, exercise, eating, climbing stairs, or walking up a hill. It may be a terrifying experience when the pain first strikes. Angina is a transient symptom in contrast to *myocardial infarction,* or heart attack, a state in which the coronary arteries are no longer able to supply any oxygen to the muscle and the muscle dies.

A typical case will illustrate the controversy prevalent today regarding coronary artery disease.

A robust, fifty-year-old married male who was vice-president of his company prided himself on his well-being. He played tennis three times a week, smoked one pack of cigarettes per day, and had a leisurely lunch each day with his cronies.

Saving time was one of his virtues; for example, in the morning he shaved and took care of his toilet needs at the same time. He drank two martinis at lunch and one with his wife in the evening.

One morning, in his usual rush to make the commuter train, he suddenly felt a tightness in his chest as he raised the garage door. The pain lasted but a few minutes. The vice-president ignored it and blamed it on indigestion. Later in the day the heaviness in his chest recurred as he climbed the stairs to the president's office. Again that night, while engaged in sexual intercourse, he suddenly experienced a terrifying sensation in his chest with tightness radiating down his left arm. He rested and the pain subsided in a few minutes.

Several days later he consulted his physician. An electrocardiogram was taken, which was normal. He felt the same pain on the bicycle during a stress test and the electrocardiogram became abnormal. His physician diagnosed angina and referred him to a cardiologist who advised cardiac catheterization and surgery. Being a modern, well-informed man, our patient sought a second opinion. Another renowned cardiologist agreed with the diagnosis of angina but thought cardiac catheterization unnecessary and surgery avoidable with proper medical treatment. What does the patient do now?

Cardiac catheterization, also referred to as *heart catheterization* or *angiography,* is a method of X-ray visualization of the heart and its blood supply, the coronary arteries, and the large blood vessels for the purpose of determining the degree and severity of the abnormalities present and the feasibility of surgical correction. Cardiac catheterization is a highly complicated diagnostic procedure involving a medical team consisting of a physician expertly trained in this procedure, assisted by nurses and X-ray and laboratory technicians. It is usually performed in a hospital.

The setting of the catheterization laboratory is akin to a science-fiction movie set: the "cath" team is garbed in heavy lead shield aprons and surgical masks and gowns. X-ray equipment, monitoring screens, TV cameras, computers, and tables with strange-looking instruments surround the electrical table on which the patient lies. Outer-space sounds of the beeping of the heart and computers intermingled with the hissing sounds of oxygen envelop the room.

An aphorism common in medicine is that there is nothing new under the sun. Cardiac catheterization was first performed in 1929 by Werner Forssmann, a twenty-five-year-old intern at a small provincial hospital north of Berlin. At the Sanders Hospital, after performing numerous experiments on dogs, he decided to do this experiment on himself.

Dr. Forssmann described the fluoroscopic procedure in his notes:

I had a mirror placed so that by looking over the top of the screen, I could see it in my thorax and upper arm. As I expected, the catheter reached the head of the humerus. I pushed the catheter in further almost to the two-foot mark. Now the mirror showed a catheter inside the heart, its tip in the right ventricle just as I had visioned it. I had some x-rays taken as a documentary experience.

The first experiment performed without anesthesia paved the road to modern heart diagnosis and surgery. The German medical establishment harassed Dr. Forssmann, claimed that he belonged in the circus, and threw him out of the hospital. Thirty-seven years later, in 1956, Dr. Forssmann was awarded the Nobel Prize.

Technique of Cardiac Catheterization

After a local anesthetic is injected, an incision is made, the artery or vein is exposed, and a long snakelike catheter is inserted, with the aid of a fluoroscope, into the thigh or the arm. It is gently passed through several large vessels, finally arriving at the heart.

The vein in the thigh or arm is punctured and entered in order to study the right side of the heart. The long, thin, flexible radiopaque plastic catheter passes into the right atrium of the heart. It is then directed through the valve which separates the right atrial chamber from the right ventricle, out of the right ventricle, and into the pulmonary artery which leads to the lungs. Meticulously, the catheter is advanced to the branches of the pulmonary artery until it is wedged in a small branch of the artery. As the catheter is advanced, blood samples are withdrawn and pressure readings are taken for the vessels and the heart vessels. There is injection of a contrast material for X-ray pictures, which are recorded. This study is called a right-sided heart catheterization, in contrast to a study of the left side of the heart, where a puncture of an artery in the thigh or arm is made. In this case the catheter is passed through the thigh artery, advancing to the aorta—the largest vessel in the body—guided through the aortic valve and into the left ventricle. The catheter is then placed into one of the coronary arteries. Contrast material is then injected, and X-ray pictures are taken.

As a rule, the procedure will last from one and a half to three hours, depending on the skill of the operator and on the ease of entry into the different structures. This invasive technique, as a rule, causes pain and discomfort, sometimes to a mild degree and sometimes more severe. For example, one of the mild discomforts is the stinging feeling of the needle prick as local anesthetic is applied. Passage of the catheter through the blood vessels is pain free, but not void of stress. Sometimes a vessel may go into spasm as the catheter is manipulated and pain will appear and fade as the vessel goes out of spasm. Sensations of skipped beats or palpitations may occur from time to time as various parts of the heart are manipulated. The patient usually feels a burning sensation when the contrast material is injected for angiography.

The type of vessel that is injected will affect the type of pain the patient feels. If the vessel is the pulmonary artery, a searing sensation will be briefly felt, sometimes quite painful. Contrast medium injected into the aorta is described generally as intense heat. When the contrast is injected into the coronary arteries, the heat may be intense, accompanied by chest pain. In all instances there is a strong urge to cough when the contrast material is injected into these vessels, and nausea and headaches sometimes accompany the pain.

The procedure is performed with the patient lying on a hard examination table which can cause patients to become stiff and cramped. If they are already suffering from chronic low-back pain, heavy sedation is needed to comfort them. Luckily, the patient needs to be rotated from time to time to get the proper angle for certain photographs, temporarily giving him some relief from lying motionless.

Some patients become distracted by the "to and fro" foreign medical language that passes between the doctors and the nurses, such as: "give him another puff," or "he has a PVC," coupled with the noises from the rapid film changer that feeds film into the X-ray unit so the sequence of pictures can be taken. With proper sedation prior to the procedure and the gentle, soft reassuring tone of the catheterization nurse, the patient is helped to endure this very difficult procedure—this procedure which summons some of the most brilliant technology of our century.

Besides the discomfort, there are risks inherent in the technique. Minor complications—ranging from inflammation of the wall of the vein to formation of clots accompanied by pain, swelling, warmth, and redness—may occur. A much more serious complication is the dislodgement of cholesterol plaques from the walls of the blood vessels which may travel and block a blood vessel supplying the brain. This may result in stroke and death. A similar blockage of a coronary artery may cause heart attack and death. Other complications, rarely seen, occur when the artery becomes blocked at the site of the catheter, the pulses disappear, and the extremities become cold—a situation requiring surgical intervention.

Allergy to injected X-ray dye and a constant fear of the operator can cause shock and death. More commonly, lesser reactions occur, such as breathing difficulties, nausea, and headaches. To forestall this complication, a small injection of the contrast medium is given prior to the procedure. The patient must also inform the physician if he has ever had a reaction before from an injected dye. As cardiac catheterization is expanding substantially, complications are decreasing. In active, experienced laboratories the death rate is approximately two per thousand, and the complication of strokes is exceedingly rare.

Fewer complications occur in institutions performing a large number of cardiac catheterizations. For example, at Emory University Hospital, where more than two thousand coronary arteriograms are done annually, the risk of serious complication is 1.5 per thousand.

The number of cardiac catheterizations performed to date would be difficult to ascertain, but a minimum of 300,000 per year would be a modest estimate. The cost of just the cardiac catheterization alone ranges from seven hundred dollars to fifteen hundred dollars per patient. This cost does not include the hospitalization and other precatheterization studies.

The physicians who perform this procedure, commonly referred to as *invasive cardiologists,* advocate it as the "gold standard" for making a proper cardiac diagnosis and often look upon noninvasive procedures with a jaundiced eye. Cardiologists who do not catheterize are called noninvasive cardiologists. All cardiologists agree that cardiac catheterization is an essential prerequisite for cardiac surgery.

Indications for Catheterization

At the Department of Radiology at Emory University School of Medicine, the following types of patients are candidates for catheterization: 1) patients who need valve surgery, 2) patients who have angina pectoris, 3) patients who have had a heart attack, 4) patients who have heart failure and an irregular heartbeat, 5) patients surviving heart arrest, and 6) asymptomatic patients who have other evidence of diseased coronary arteries and numerous other indications that need not be listed.

Invasive cardiologists claim that the only method that can accurately diagnose the presence and severity of coronary artery disease is cardiac catheterization.

It is not fair to the patient to diagnose this disease on clinical grounds alone, as sometimes the diagnosis is wrong and the patient suffers undue hardship and expense. For example, the patient may find difficulties in career advancement, or in obtaining a job or life insurance. Airplane pilots are permanently excluded from their profession.

Unfortunately, too often the patient carries the diagnosis of angina along with his bottle of pills, when, in reality, he may be suffering from a gastrointestinal disorder, such as a hiatal her-

nia. The latter is a great simulator of heart disease. So confus-
ing are these two conditions that, in the not too distant past,
patients died of "indigestion" when, in reality, they suffered a
heart attack.

The Opposing View

Diagnosis and severity of angina has been accurately made
for two hundred years on clinical grounds alone. More recently
diagnosis has been confirmed with the cardiac stress test and
another examination, called *nuclear scanning,* without the need
for cardiac catheterization.

Any diagnostic procedure that can endanger the life of the
patient must be carefully weighed and evaluated. The procedure must justify the results that will be obtained. Any diagnostic procedure that can cause death, great discomfort, a string of
serious complications, and is costly as well must be soberly scru-
tinized. The noninvasive cardiologist is anxious to achieve a
precise diagnosis and outline a suitable plan, but not if the
diagnostic procedure is worse than the disease.

An astute, well-trained cardiologist needs little more than a
keen ear and an intelligent brain to diagnose a heart ailment.
Some excellent cardiologists are capable of making a judicious
diagnosis merely by palpating the patient's chest, "feeling the
murmurs." Their hands become as sensitive as their ears.

These noninvasive procedures are relatively inexpensive and
can be performed outside a hospital setting. For example, it is
no longer necessary to have a patient undergo cardiac catheterization to diagnose a rheumatic heart ailment. Using *echocardiography,* or *sonar,* a fascinating and intriguing method of vi-
sualizing the heart by sound waves, the structure of the valves
can be delineated with a moderate degree of accuracy, and an
estimation of the severity of obstruction or flow of blood
through these valves can be determined. The cost of echocardiography is but a fraction of what cardiac catheterization costs.
Furthermore, echocardiography can be repeated hundreds of
times without any discomfort to the patient.

Other modern techniques, such as nuclear angiography, can determine the function of the heart without penetrating the heart. With the recent advent of two-dimensional echocardiography, a step further is taken away from the cardiac catheterization table, as now the heart can be visualized as a moving structure. Echocardiography, in one sense, is even more accurate in determining heart abnormalities, such as tumors.

Cardiac catheterization should be performed if angina is not responsive to maximum medical treatment, disabling the patient and making his life unbearable. It is in this instance that cardiac catheterization is needed to determine the extent of narrowing of the coronary arteries and whether surgery will be able to correct the abnormality.

Echocardiography does not allow visualization of coronary arteries with our present technique. On the other hand, if angina is of a mild nature, readily controlled with our new medical treatment, and surgery is not a consideration, catheterization adds little to the management of the patient.

When the physician suspects that the patient has severe narrowing of the coronary arteries in spite of moderate symptoms of angina, it also is necessary to perform an angiogram. A very abnormal electrocardiogram or a blatantly abnormal stress test may cause the physician to suspect that the main coronary artery is stenosed. Death from a severely occluded main coronary artery occurs at the rate of 30 to 60 percent per year. Fortunately, main artery disease occurs in only 10 to 16 percent of patients with angina.

Proponents of cardiac catheterization advocate that the patient's coronary arteries be studied after a heart attack in most instances. Again, it is the opinion of noninvasive cardiologists not to submit the patient to this procedure unless he develops angina after the heart attack that disables him or he does not respond to medical treatment. Then surgery is contemplated.

Sometimes patients themselves insist on an angiogram. For example, when chest pain is present and the physician finds all tests are normal (electrocardiogram, stress test, and newer tests like the thallium stress test and echocardiogram), and the patient "wants to know," an angiogram is likely to be performed.

If a physician discovers a heart murmur during a routine examination on an asymptomatic patient, as a rule cardiac catheterization is not required for the physician to arrive at a proper diagnosis. With the availability of echocardiography and other noninvasive cardiac techniques, the origin of a murmur can be outlined. Unless a congenital heart condition is found in an asymptomatic patient, early surgery may be indicated and must be preceded by proper invasive studies.

Some centers perform angiography in asymptomatic patients after finding abnormal stress tests, irregular rhythms, or hearts enlarged from unknown cause. With our newer techniques catheterization can be deferred.

There should be no hesitation on the part of the physician or the patient to encourage a second opinion. Preferably, the second opinion should be obtained from a noninvasive cardiologist.

Sometimes the family physician, faced with the discovery of a heart murmur or other cardiac abnormality, rightfully refers the patient to a cardiologist. When the cardiologist is also a "catheter man," he will not be opposed to suggest an angiogram to firm up his diagnosis. A second opinion is warranted if the patient is hesitant about undergoing this procedure.

The primary goal of medical practice is to help the patient. Doctors who advocate angiography sincerely do it for the benefit of the patient. It is essential, however, that the patient realizes that there are other available alternatives that yield a great deal of information regarding their condition. It is indisputable that indications for cardiac catheterizations are shrinking as more and more brilliant technology becomes available. In the not too distant future, catheterization laboratories will likely become less widespread, the number of procedures will diminish, and a marked increase of noninvasive cardiologists will characterize the world of cardiac practice.

CORONARY BYPASS SURGERY
Surgical Opinion

For two hundred years, the medical man has been grappling with the problem of angina, ever since Heberden's original description in 1768:

> . . . a disorder of the breast marked with strong peculiar symptoms, considerable for the kind of danger belonging to it and not extremely rare, of which I do not recall any mention among medical authors, the seat of it and sense of strangling and anxiety with which it is attended make it being called angina pectoris. Those who are afflicted with it are seized while they are walking and more particularly when they walk soon after eating, with a painful and most disagreeable sensation in the breast which seems as if it would take their life away, if it were to increase or continue; the moment they stand still all this uneasiness vanishes.

Its cause, as well as its treatment, even up to this day, remains controversial. Volumes of paper and millions of dollars of research later, and the etiology of coronary arteriosclerosis remains speculative. Forms of treatment are prescribed with some proven basis, but mostly on sheer speculation and epidemiological evidence. Strict dietary regulations are recommended, taking away some of the fundamental foodstuffs that we all adore, as cheese, eggs and meat; exercises are prescribed to patients who never exercised before and despise it; medications like nitroglycerin are prescribed, which can cause such side effects as intolerable headaches, while the "miracle drug propranolol" can make the poor soul chronically fatigued, sometimes impotent, curtail his exercise tolerance, but can also relieve his angina. But at what expense! In spite of strict dietary programs, weight reduction, job changes, psychiatric consultations, and lengthy intolerable drug usage, the patient still may die suddenly or sustain a heart attack (myocardial infarction).

For almost two hundred years the medical treatment of this condition remained unchanged. All sorts of potions, chest rub-

bings, spas, and purgatives were devised. In the 1800s Sir
Thomas L. Bunton, of London, discovered liquid nitroglycerin, called amyl nitrate, an effective method of relieving patients with angina. To this very day nitroglycerin remains the
main therapeutic agent. During one of the authors' training
periods, in 1950, patients were counseled to reduce their activities, rest as much as possible, and take nitroglycerin. The
angina patient became a cardiac cripple. The simplest activities—combing his hair, dressing, eating, arising from a chair—
would be accompanied by severe pain.

Scientists have long understood that if the blocked arteries
could be bypassed, or new channels built into the heart with a
fresh supply of oxygen, then the anginal symptoms would be
eradicated. In 1935 Dr. Claude Beck attempted to connect a
new blood supply into a patient's heart. The first surgeon credited for actually creating new blood vessels was Dr. Arthur
Vineberg, who, in 1950, devised a method of implanting the
artery into the heart and bypassing the narrow coronary arteries. The operation had some degree of success, but the new
arteries swiftly became occluded. Finally, in 1967, Dr. Renée
Favallaro and Dr. W. Dudley Johnson devised the bypass operation currently used today.

The exciting era of coronary bypass surgery had begun. Patients who were completely disabled, resistant to even the more
modern forms of medical treatment, finally had their relief.
From a meager several thousand operative procedures, there
was an increase to seventy-five thousand operations performed
per year. Surgery became a blessing for the individual who was
disabled from angina, as the sufferers had an 80 to 90 percent
chance of being symptom free. This busy enterprise is a highly
lucrative one, costing the public one billion dollars per year.

Techniques of Coronary Artery Bypass Surgery

The procedure consists of taking a vein from the leg or an
artery from the chest, bypassing the useless obstructed artery,

and creating a new path for the flow of blood and oxygen. The vein or artery now functions like the artery it replaced. Any of the coronary arteries can be bypassed (left, right, circumflex, etc.), providing there are normal vessels to make the hookups. If the vessel below the obstruction is very narrowed, no correction is possible.

The heart needs a continual supply of blood and the oxygen it carries. With exercise, more blood and oxygen are needed. Angina usually is present when the degree of arterial narrowing is greater than 90 percent. However, a 75 percent reduction can also cause angina if the subject is exercising or just walking briskly. If the heartbeat suddenly increases, as during sexual intercourse, angina can also occur. Some patients may suffer no angina at all, even with critical narrowing of the arteries, but sustain heart damage silently, sometimes referred to as a silent heart attack.

Under ideal conditions, with an experienced cardiac surgeon in a reputable medical center, the death rate of the surgery is in the vicinity of 1 to 5 percent. The overall statistic for the anginal symptom being improved or eliminated is 80 to 100 percent of patients, or an expected 20 percent failure rate can result from surgery, which means the angina has not improved or even may become worse. The reappearance of angina results from the graft becoming occluded.

If surgery is not performed on the symptomatic diseased artery, the death rate per year is as follows: If one vessel is critically narrowed, the death rate per year is in the vicinity of 4 percent; if two vessels are diseased, death occurs between 7 and 10 percent per year; if three vessels are diseased, the mortality rate increases markedly in a five-year rate without surgery of 50 percent. If the left main vessel is critically diseased, the mortality is 30 to 40 percent per year.

The medical man gives temporary relief to the patient and a false sense of being well as he trudges through life with arteries that are incompatible with a normal existence and which can carry him away at any moment. Giving medications to control angina, in some sense, is like giving aspirin for fever; the illness carries on although the symptom is temporarily alleviated, but the pathology is not corrected.

It is pitiful to watch the patient with angina becoming a cardiac cripple, popping nitroglycerin in his mouth before a leisurely stroll to forestall that "old feeling" in his chest. Prior to engaging in copulation, he must scurry around for the nitro pill to place under his tongue ten minutes before the act, while his partner looks on with fear and dismay. Notices of famed actors sustaining heart attacks during conjugal unions come to mind, and sex becomes a terrifying act for the partners. Many times the sexual life of the couple comes to an end. The activities of the ardent tennis player, the ski enthusiast, or the jogger are suddenly cut short with this illness, and for them life lacks richness. Coronary artery bypass surgery can put the tennis player back on the court, the skier back on the slope, and the lover back to sexual activity. Is it not the quality of life that matters and not the quantity?

When the left main artery is obstructed, death is imminent in close to 60 percent of the patients studied. In a recent Veteran's Administration randomized study, survival for one year for a medically treated group was compared with that for a surgically treated group. Sixty-eight percent of patients treated medically were alive at one year as compared with 88 percent in those who had had bypass surgery. In a study at the Cleveland Clinic, patients who had three-vessel disease showed similar results to those with left main disease. Surgery prolonged life in surgically treated patients as compared with medically treated patients.

The indications for surgery are firmly established in patients who are suffering from intractable angina. These patients will benefit from bypass surgery 80 to 90 percent of the time—almost complete relief of symptoms. Surgeons advocate that surgery be performed if two vessels are 75 percent stenosed, whether the patient is symptomatic or not. If one blood vessel is found to be severely diseased, some surgeons advocate that bypass be performed on this vessel, even if the patient suffers only from mild angina.

Another indication for performing bypass surgery is when young patients suffer myocardial infarction; surgery should then be performed a reasonable time after this event, especially if a grossly abnormal stress test is found, even if the patient is asymptomatic. Also, patients who develop a sudden chaotic rhythm, called *ventricular fibrillation,* should have an arteriogram and surgery. Ventricular fibrillation is an irregular rhythm that precedes death unless the condition is properly treated.

Age alone should not be a determinant in performing bypass surgery. A seventy-five-year-old man disabled with angina can be operated on, especially if he is an active person with no renal disease or brain ailment.

When the medical man provides us with a form of treatment that fully controls coronary artery disease, prevents sudden death, and has a means of preventing the illness in the first place, then surgery can go by the wayside. Until that time, which hopefully will be in the near future, surgery is a reasonable answer to the dilemma of coronary artery disease.

The Medical Point of View

There are, at the present time, three major indications for performing bypass surgery. Those patients who continue to have severe angina in spite of maximal treatment with nitrates and propranolol, control of hypertension, cessation of cigarette smoking, and weight reduction are categorized as intractable angina sufferers and are candidates for angiography, and, if possible, bypass surgery.

When the left main artery is stenosed by greater than 75 percent, or three vessels are stenosed and the patient is asymptomatic, there is full agreement among surgical colleagues on

the need to operate. If, after the patient has sustained a myocardial infarction, his angina continues in spite of excellent
treatment, bypass surgery is also indicated.

As for coronary bypass surgery prolonging life in patients
with two-vessel disease or one-vessel disease, there are inadequate data to warrant this conclusion. Before a patient and his
physician make a decision to have bypass surgery, the following
facts should be presented: 10 percent of the inserted new
grafts become occluded immediately after surgery and another
10 to 20 percent during the first year. Thereafter there is a
continued rate of 2 percent per year of occlusion. By five years
after the operation, one-third or more of grafts will be occluded and one-third of the patients will have at least one occluded graft. Newer evidence suggests that, at the end of six to
seven years, 60 percent of the grafts are occluded, which means
that angina then reappears. It also appears that surgery may
actually accelerate the arteriosclerosis of the nongrafted arteries, but this is still speculative.

Another disheartening finding is that approximately 30 percent of patients whose grafts are occluded do not have the
reappearance of angina—a fact suggesting a placebo effect in
surgery. In 1968 a Swedish study demonstrated that 50 percent
of patients with occluded bypass grafts had the same improvement in their symptoms and exercise tolerance as those patients
whose grafts were patent. The results of these cases also
strongly imply a surgical placebo effect.

Placebo effect, or psychological relief from an ineffective form
of physiological treatment, has been known to medicine since
antiquity, from the famed sugar pill to the sterile needle injection and a convincing doctor's power of suggestion. Before
bypass surgery was devised, Dr. Gray Diamond and his associ-
ates showed that many patients with angina pectoris experienced significant relief from symptoms following a sham operation consisting merely of a skin incision on the chest. The
greater the patient's incentive to get well, the more likely he
will experience a favorable placebo effect.

In the majority of patients who have undergone bypass surgery, benefits occur because of increased blood flow to the heart. Surgeons claim that bypass surgery not only relieves angina but also improves the function of the heart. An equal wealth of data reports that only a minority of patients operated on improve their cardiac function.

The cause of arteriosclerosis is unknown. Neither diet, exercise, nor bypass surgery alters its progression. If the patient is willing to accept bypass surgery as a temporary form of treatment which gives him relief 80 to 90 percent of the time, with the 60 to 70 percent possibility of symptoms recurring at the end of seven years, then, by all means, that patient should go ahead and have surgery. Furthermore, he should realize that the operation will not prolong his life unless the left main artery is diseased or all three vessels are clogged.

Ten times more surgery is performed in the United States than in Europe. It is not known whether Americans are doing too much surgery or Europeans too little. The causes cited for the Europeans doing less surgery are lack of special nursing care, stricter medical criteria, and lack of facilities. One British cardiologist stated that "For you chaps in America, it becomes an economic necessity. We don't have such a need for the operation and prefer to wait for its effectiveness." Dr. G. Braunwald remarked: "The financial integrity of all medical centers has become dependent on the continued flow of patients for aorto-coronary bypass grafting."

Since there are four million or more people suffering from coronary artery disease, it is reasonable to assume that bypass surgery is here to stay. To determine the long-term efficacy of this operation, as compared with medical treatment, studies are being conducted throughout the United States. These studies are essential lest we continue doing vast numbers of surgery whose effectiveness is unproven. (An allied example is Dr. William Halsted's experience in 1894 when he recommended radical mastectomy as the treatment of choice for cancer of the breast. Eighty-three years later this operation is being challenged as a life-prolonging procedure. Halsted's type of conventional radical surgical operation is rapidly diminishing in popularity.)

A new method of treating coronary arteries is now being tested. The method, called *percutaneous transluminal coronary angioplasty,* consists of passing a specialized catheter into the obstructed artery and compressing the arteriosclerotic material into the vessel wall. The procedure originated in Zurich, Switzerland, and is currently being tried in this country. It is too soon to draw any conclusions about the benefits of this nonsurgical procedure, but it may offer a reasonable alternative to bypass surgery.

The current collective opinion of many cardiologists on the results of coronary bypass surgery is as follows:

1. It does not prolong life unless the left main vessel is diseased or three vessels are critically narrowed.
2. Angina is markedly improved or eliminated in 80 to 90 percent of cases in the first year.
3. The definitive cure will be prevention of the disease in the first place.

VALVULAR SURGERY

"Rheumatic fever licks the joints and bites the heart." So went the saying of older clinicians. When rheumatic fever "bites the heart," it attacks the valves, which may leave the patient with a "rheumatic heart," the outstanding symptom of heart murmurs, and later a terrifying heart disability that, in many instances, only surgery can cure.

Today, rheumatic fever is becoming rare in our Western society, though it is still prevalent in the poorer nations of the world, such as Okinawa, the Philippines, Korea, and Vietnam. In the United States it is uncommon to hear of a young person with a rheumatic heart and valvular disease, unless it is congenital. Most of the patients seen today are forty or fifty years old, in comparison with the average in the Far East or Philippines, where the abnormalities appear in the twenties or thirties. Arteriosclerosis is the major cause of aortic valve disease in our society.

The Anatomy and Pathology of the Mitral and Aortic Valves

The mitral valve has two leaflets, and it separates the left atrial cavity from the left ventricle, permitting the flow of blood from the upper chamber to the lower chamber. This valve is called mitral because of its resemblance to a mitre, a headdress worn by bishops. The aortic valve, which looks like a bird's nest, has three leaflets and guides the blood flow from the left side of the heart into the aorta and out toward the rest of the body. The mitral valve is more commonly afflicted than the aortic valve.

When diseased, these valves, because of inflammation and a progressive destructive process, either cannot close or open. This is called insufficiency, or *stenosis*. When the valve is markedly narrowed, the blood cannot flow forward and the blood backs up into the lungs. When the valve cannot close, the blood flows forward, and some of the blood also returns back through the valve. The only symptom of having a diseased valve may be the fortuitous finding of a heart murmur during a routine examination.

Symptoms of a Diseased Valve

In the beginning, as these valves become abnormal, symptoms appear, consisting of fatigue, shortness of breath after exertion, and irregular heartbeats. If the disease progresses, the patient may suffer increasing shortness of breath at rest, with swelling of ankles and fluid accumulating in the lungs and other parts of the body. This is referred to as *congestive heart failure,* which indicates that the valves have caused a backing up of blood, diminishing the ability of the heart to pump efficiently. Eventually, in spite of the medical treatment, the patient succumbs to his illness unless the valve is replaced.

Prior to the availability of echocardiography and cardiac catheterization, it was pure speculation on the part of the physician which determined which valve was diseased. During the authors' student days, when the professor pointed out a heart murmur, his word would be taken as final. Later, when echocardiography and cardiac catheterization came on the scene, his findings could be confirmed.

MITRAL STENOSIS

When the mitral valve becomes narrowed by disease, we speak of mitral stenosis. It may take ten years from the time of the attack of rheumatic fever and the actual hearing of a heart murmur. Another ten years may pass before symptoms are noted. This is not the case in areas like Vietnam, Alaska, or Malaysia, where severe mitral stenosis may develop at a young age. Patients with mitral stenosis have symptoms that begin to progress gradually over several years, becoming aggravated during pregnancy and physical stress.

THE AORTIC VALVE

As a result of congenital deformities, rheumatic fever, or aging, the aortic valve with its three leaflets can become destroyed and narrowed. The consequence of this narrowing is called aortic stenosis. Symptoms of this valvular disease may appear suddenly, at a much later age, in contrast with mitral valve disease symptoms, which can have a gradual onset. Some patients may notice chest pain classical of angina even though their coronary arteries are normal. Other symptoms include shortness of breath, fainting, irregular heartbeat. Sudden death can also occur.

The murmur of aortic stenosis may be so faint that even an experienced physician can ignore its significance and treat the patient for coronary artery disease. The patient becomes worse and may die suddenly. Proper testing with echocardiography and cardiac catheterization and subsequent valve replacement can save and prolong a life.

Surgery of Mitral and Aortic Valves

In the early 1940s surgery on the mitral valve was performed by a rather simple technique of widening the orifice with a finger or knife. This technique, called *mitral commissurotomy*, or finger dilatation, is still used in surgery when the valve is freely movable and not thickened and calcified. Not all valves could be treated in that fashion and surgical replacement of the heart valves was inevitable. Cadaveric valves were placed and artificial valves were devised.

In 1949 Dr. R. Denton was the first to place a polyethylon prosthesis, but the first complete excision replacement of the mitral valve took place on March 10, 1960.

Currently, one-half of the valves replaced are derived from the pig, called porcine xenographs. This valve is fabricated from natural aortic valve procured from commercial slaughterhouses as fresh tissue. After transfer to the factory the valve is trimmed, tanned in a special solution, and stored ready for use. This new valve has the advantage of not causing clots, and thus decreases the need for anticoagulation. However, its durability is not yet known.

The longer that the valvular disease is present with obstructive symptoms, the weaker the heart and the worse the prognosis at surgery. The mortality rate from valve surgery is in the vicinity of 3 to 10 percent. The major regret of the surgeon is that the patient arrives too late.

If the patient is asymptomatic and shows evidence from cardiac catheterization studies of severe aortic stenosis, some surgeons and cardiologists favor replacement of the valve. Preferably, surgery should be done on patients who are only slightly limited in their physical activity. Once the patient is

severely disabled, his prognosis becomes much worse. If the
aortic valve is shown to be severely narrowed, then, even
though the patient is mildly symptomatic, surgery will be recommended. A recent example comes to mind.

J. B., a seventy-five-year-old sturdy-looking man, developed
"angina" of recent onset. His family physician prescribed appropriate drugs for this condition and advised him to "slow
down." J. B. was not the sort of man to slow down, so instead
he went to see another physician, a cardiologist, who suspected
aortic stenosis, which was confirmed with echocardiography
and cardiac catheterization. J. B.'s arteries were as normal as
those of an eighteen-year-old, but the valve was calcified and
narrowed. The valve was replaced with a pig's valve and the patient became symptom free.

In the case of severe aortic stenosis, or narrowing of the aortic valve, death can be sudden and unexpected. When symptoms start to appear, such as chest pain, dizziness, abnormal
heartbeats, or shortness of breath, valve replacement must be
performed, as the progression is swift and relentless. The same
could be said if the valve is incompetent, also called *aortic
regurgitation.*

The surgeons point to thirty years' experience with valve
surgery, which, for the most part, has had excellent results.
However, in the case of aortic stenosis, without surgery, the expected death rate is approximately 15 to 30 percent per year
once symptoms of the valve disorder appear. In the case of mitral stenosis there is a much longer period of survival time
without surgery, as the symptoms take longer to surface. Today
surgery of aortic stenosis has a survival rate of 85 percent after
four years, whereas ten years ago it was 35 percent. Why, then,
not operate?

The Medical Point of View

It is the clinical evaluation of the patient which will determine when surgery is indicated. Surgeons will have a tendency
to take the catheterization data, representing the anatomical

structural abnormality of the valve, as indications for surgery.

In the case of a stenotic valve when the patient has minimal symptoms, surgery should be deferred as long as possible. It is true that early surgery may bring better results, but it would be difficult for most cardiologists to recommend surgery when the patient has minimal symptoms.

Cardiologists fully agree that once aortic stenosis presents with symptoms such as dizziness, chest pain, and shortness of breath, surgery should be performed; likewise, in the case of the valve being incompetent (aortic regurgitation), as symptoms advance, surgery should also be performed at once. When an irregular beat results from a stenotic valve, this is not an indication to perform surgery, as the irregular beat may continue even after surgery.

The patient should not accept valve replacement until a thorough history and physical examination have been performed. Studies should include a cardiac stress test (except in aortic stenosis) to define the actual moment and severity of the disability, and an echocardiogram to complement the cardiac catheterization. Sometimes cardiac catheterization cannot give the total picture of the degree of disease of the valve. An operation that is performed too soon may not be beneficial to the patient. On the other hand, surgery performed on far advanced heart disease, when the heart is severely damaged, has a poor result and high mortality rate.

Age is not a deterrent for valve replacement. For example, in the case of severe aortic stenosis (chest pain, shortness of breath with slight exertion) and normal coronary arteries, surgery can render the remainder of the patient's life comfortable. On the other hand, in the case of advanced mitral insufficiency, newer enthusiastic medical management is used to keep the patient in a state of well-being. Surgery often is used too early or too late in this condition.

In these circumstances it is wise to obtain a second opinion from another cardiologist in order to discuss alternative forms of treatment.

The patient must also know that there is a 5 to 10 percent mortality rate from replacement of the valve and that he lives with the constant threat of complications from the artificial valve. To mention but a few: infection of the prosthetic valve, anemia secondary to the valve macerating red blood cells, and, the most dreaded complication, clots passing from a valve to the vital organs of the body. This latter complication, called *pulmonary embolism,* is, to a large part, brought under control with a blood-thinning substance called Coumadin. A lifetime commitment to anticoagulation is necessary. Uncontrolled bleeding, the complication resulting from anticoagulation drugs, occurs at a rate of 5 to 10 percent per year.

Employing the porcine xenograft valve in elderly patients is the present procedure, as this type of valve does not appear to cause clots and anticoagulation is generally not needed. It is not used in the younger patient because the durability of this valve is not known.

Valvular surgery is one of the miracles of this century. Patients who once might have been totally disabled all their lives and succumbed early are now living normal existences. However, the indications must be precise, the surgeon experienced, and surgery done in a hospital where many operations are performed rather than in one which does only an occasional valve replacement, for in this latter situation the mortality rate will be higher than 5 to 10 percent.

PACEMAKERS

At the racquet club in Palm Springs, a seventy-four-year-old gentleman has just finished playing the second set of tennis singles when he suddenly begins to feel dizzy and weak. It is eleven o'clock in the morning and the day is oppressively hot, but he continues to play until the moment when he collapses and stares blankly at the bright sky. His doctor examines him and finds that he has a slow pulse rate of 35.

Another person, a female, who is sitting with her friends,

playing cards, and losing bitterly, begins to feel faint. She has had these weak spells off and on for years and has been told by her physician that they were due to nervousness. Other physicians have told her that not enough blood is reaching her brain, and still others state that she has a pinched nerve in her neck. A cardiologist finally diagnosed a peculiar heart rhythm that causes her heart to slow down suddenly and sometimes actually to stop.

A truck driver in Indianapolis has a near-fatal accident as he collapses while driving his truck, which crashes over an embankment.

All three patients have one thing in common: their hearts suddenly slow, not delivering enough oxygen to their brains, causing them to become dizzy and collapse. All three have a pacemaker implanted and become totally symptom free.

A high-strung fifty-eight-year-old female was once told by a physician that she had a heart murmur, heart disease, and angina, although her electrocardiogram had been normal. She, too, had had episodes of fainting and dizzy spells. After reading in some health magazines about the miracles of pacemakers, she approached her physician and told him what her problem was.

"I know I need a pacemaker, Doctor, because I always run a slow pulse." Her pulse was 68.

She did not have adequate testing and documentation before a pacemaker was inserted. Several months later her dizziness and fainting episodes reappeared.

These four cases demonstrate the use of pacemakers. In the United States alone there are approximately 200,000 people living with implanted pacemakers. It has been estimated that in the next ten years another 100,000 will have their hearts paced by an artificial internal device. The average pacemaker recipient is seventy-two years of age and has a life expectancy of twelve years, with 40 percent more women alive than men. Eighty percent of the pacer patient population is over fifty-five. It has been estimated that one out of every three hundred persons over fifty-five years of age, or one out of every fifteen hundred of the total population, carries an implanted pacemaker.

Physiology of Pacemakers

All human beings are born with their own internal pacemakers. It is because we have our own pacemakers that the heart is able to contract normally, pumping 10 pints of blood every day along a route of seventy-five thousand miles to three trillion cells. This specialized electrical system generates the impulse for cardiac contraction. It originates in special cells called pacemaker cells, which are grouped at the uppermost part of the heart, called the SA node, and sends signals through special tracts to another point, called the AV node. It then divides into branches, supplying the right and left ventricles. These electrical currents flow smoothly but occasionally are interrupted or stimulated by a variety of agents, such as coffee, alcohol, excitement, cigarette smoking, and too little oxygen in normal individuals. The interruption, or the extra impulse, causes the sensation of a skipped beat, an extra beat, or a feeling of "my heart turning in my chest," referred to as palpitations.

The transmission of this electricity through the branches makes the heart contract normally between 60 to 85 beats per minute. The pulse rate may vary from individual to individual. Some people may have normal pulse beats of 45 and 50 all their lives. Athletes tend to have lower pulse beats. Children have a faster pulse beat than young adults and the aged have a slower pulse beat than children.

The History of Pacemakers

In 1872 the first heart was paced by Dr. Guillaume-Benjamin Armand Duchenne. He used rhythmic electrical stimulation of the chest in order to resuscitate patients who collapsed. His technique consisted of two electrodes, one placed on the patient's body, the other stimulating electrode held by Dr. Duchenne in his hand. Duchenne actually resuscitated a twenty-year-old female whose heart went into a complete chaotic irregular beat called ventricular fibrillation. The woman was successfully resuscitated more than one hundred years ago.

The earliest pacemakers consisted of electrodes with a power source, attached to the skin, but, as you might expect, this was highly unsatisfactory, as they caused severe burns. In November of 1956 the first electrodes were placed into the heart muscle by Dr. Henry Bahanson at Johns Hopkins University. Walter Lilleihi and his team then continued work on the placement of artificial pacemakers.

Indications for Pacemaker Use

When the conduction becomes completely interrupted and the ventricles beat independently from the rest of the heart, we speak of a *complete heart block*. The pulse may then be 35 or less. Numerous other conditions arise, termed *partial heart block, complete heart block, anterior hemi-block*, etc. In some of these instances the heart is not only beating slowly, it may periodically stop and then restart. This sudden slowing of the heart to a pulse rate below 40, or the sudden arrest of the heart, can cause a patient to collapse, have dizzy spells, fainting spells, and a variety of neurological symptoms ranging from double vision to headaches and seizures. Chronic fatigue, poor exercise abilities, and, unfortunately, on occasion sudden death may result. Therefore, when the pacemaker fails—because of a heart attack or sclerosis, infection, injuries, and so forth—then an artificial pacemaker must be inserted, a pacemaker that will now take over the job of stimulating the heart.

It must be fully documented that the patient does indeed have a heart block with a resultant slow pulse or episodes of cardiac standstill. Casual listening to the heartbeat and examining the patient will not provide sufficient evidence of the patient's need for a pacemaker. Most centers throughout the United States require a cardiologist to confirm the diagnosis with appropriate testing before referring the patient to the surgeon.

Pacemakers should not be inserted unless proper care can be provided. Surveillance systems needed to check the workings of the pacemaker range from simple periodic monitoring of an electrocardiographic rhythm strip to comprehensive clinics providing detailed study. It is possible to test the competency of the pacemaker over the telephone. If pacemaker surveillance cannot be provided, the patient should either get another surgeon or refuse to have a pacemaker. It needs to be re-emphasized that the biggest problem of pacemaker insertion is trying to document that dizziness, fainting, or weak spells are caused by the heart and not by something else. The patient must be certain that the surgeon is an expert in pacing; he must have an understanding of the electrophysiology, electrocardiography, and surgical techniques, and be fully aware of the various pacing failures and management of complications.

Description of Pacemaker

The pacemaker is a small unit, about the size of a cigarette package (we apologize for that dirty word), containing batteries that produce impulses to make the heart beat. A long electrode connects the battery to the right side of the heart. The pacemaker is preset for a particular pulse rate.

The earliest pacemakers were inserted by actually opening the chest wall and implanting them into the heart. By 1965 pacemakers were inserted by threading them through an arm or shoulder vein; going through the chest wall was no longer necessary. Pacemakers are still implanted through the chest when the chest is already opened during heart surgery. The pacemaker is then placed in the right side of the heart.

The Current Technique

Under fluoroscopic control, an opening is made in the vein and the electrode is passed into the right side of the heart to a wedged position. The electrode is attached to the battery, which is placed in a skin pocket constructed in front of the chest. The anatomic and functional position is confirmed with the fluoroscope, and, for the next twenty-four to forty-eight hours the patient is monitored by electrocardiogram to be certain that the electrode does not get displaced, as it does in 5 to 10 percent of patients. A chest X ray is taken at that time to confirm the position of the pacemaker. These pacemakers are called permanent pacemakers, in contradistinction to temporary pacemakers or temporary pacing, which is frequently used in a coronary care unit when a very slow heartbeat occurs, as sometimes after a myocardial infarction.

Types of Pacemakers

The simplest pacemaker fires at a fixed automatic rate. The impulses pace the heart at a predetermined rate anywhere from 70 to 75 beats per minute. In making a decision about whether a pacemaker should be inserted, the patient should also know that several types of batteries are currently in use. The classical workhorse of the industry was the mercury zinc cell, which has waned in popularity. Its recent average life span has been about thirty-eight months, but some have lasted five years. Now in use are lithium cells and regular isotope or nuclear cells.

The nuclear pacemakers first implanted in humans in 1970 have now been released by the Nuclear Regulatory Commission for general use in the United States. The battery is designed to last ten years or more. Plutonium nuclear pacemakers took a long time to be approved because of the opposition of environmentalists who feared that if the casing were not strong enough, plutonium would spread through the environment. The casing also had to be bulletproof in case of a gunshot wound. In addition, the housing of the pacemaker had to be able to withstand heat. One crematorium in New Jersey used such high temperatures that the shell of the unit was melted.

Plutonium pacemakers today are made to withstand all these insults. Lithium-powered pacemakers last for six to eight years and newer ones that may last longer are on the way. The basic goal is to find a pacemaker that will last a lifetime.

The type of pacemakers that should be used is outlined below:

1. Patients with a limited life expectancy should choose a pacemaker with either a mercury, zinc, or lithium battery.
2. For middle-aged patients, a lithium pacemaker or, preferably, a nuclear unit should be used to ensure long functional life to the pacemaker.

Complications and Problems of the Pacemaker

1) Malposition—the pacemaker electrode is placed in the wrong place or it gets dislodged from its position on the right side of the heart. 2) The sensitivity is set incorrectly and the heart is over- or under-stimulated. 3) There may be hemorrhages at the site of the pocket of the battery. 4) Rarely, fractures may occur at the wires in the heart or at the vein entrance, at the connector, or in the free wire. 5) Unfortunately, sometimes the pacemaker itself may be defective after it is inserted, or the battery runs down prematurely. This is why surveillance of the pacemaker is so important.

The patient must also recognize that the unit itself, or the battery, will be placed underneath the skin, with a bulge evident. Females, rightfully, will be concerned about their appearance in a bathing suit or with a low décolletage. Surgeons will take into consideration the cosmetic needs of the individual patient.

When the physician advises the insertion of a pacemaker, the patient must, in turn, respond: "How do you know?" We strongly urge a second opinion if the patient's heart had not been monitored for at least a twenty-four-hour period. The monitoring system can be accomplished by a device called the

Holter monitor, which the patient carries as a sling over his shoulder with electrodes attached on the surface of his body. The patient keeps an accurate record of the times when he feels dizzy or weak or has other symptoms, which is later corroborated by the tape of the recording of the patient's heart. If it indeed demonstrates episodes of complete standstill of the heart or very slow pulse beats while the patient is symptomatic, then the pacemaker should be inserted. Monitoring with a continuous electrocardiogram in a hospital for several days is equally good, if not better. A cardiac stress test may also be helpful in revealing any irregularities of the heart.

A very slow pulse rate of 40 or 38 in a completely asymptomatic patient may not necessarily warrant a pacemaker, unless it occurs with a patient who definitely has an abnormal heart, as secondary to a myocardial infarction, infection, or rheumatic heart disease. In these situations a pacemaker might be considered prophylactically. Although pacemakers do not prevent heart attacks or inhibit hardening of the arteries, they are critically involved with the electrical conduction of the heart.

STRESS TESTING

It is appropriate to spend some time in a book of this kind on stress testing, as this procedure is included in the cardiovascular diagnostic workup that occurs before the patient has surgery. In addition, headlines in the press, stemming from the medical literature, dispute the necessity and value of stress tests. This controversy came to a head only recently when President Carter collapsed during a foot race; later it was learned that he had not undergone a stress test. His physician, Rear Admiral William Lukash, the White House doctor, stated that as the president had no symptoms of heart trouble, it led him to conclude that it was not needed. Lukash stated that President Carter had none of the risk factors, such as hypertension, diabetes, insufficient exercise, and high blood fats, and the accuracy of the test would be of limited value.

Before entering further into this extraordinary controversy, a brief glimpse of what cardiac stress testing is and what information is furnished by this procedure will be described.

The principle of the exercise stress test, or cardiac stress testing, is based on the physiological response that results when the individual is asked to exercise either on a bicycle or a treadmill, the two apparatuses currently used to test a patient's endurance. Historically, the Chinese, Romans, and Greeks used the treadmill for irrigation construction over two thousand years ago. In 1818 William Cubitt, a British civil engineer, designed an elongated stepping wheel on which dozens of prisoners could work side by side, a form of punishment regarded as a cruel, inhuman, and unhealthy practice. Today we pay a sizable amount to undergo this same type of testing.

Physiological and metabolic response of humans to muscular exercise has been performed for decades. As early as 1857 exercise testing was performed to determine capabilities for swimming, rowing, and horseback riding. It was in the early 1940s when cardiologists realized that an electrocardiogram taken with the patient lying comfortably on the examining table was not an accurate picture of the events that take place in the heart. The circumstances that occur at rest are physiologically different from those that occur with effort. The late Dr. Arthur Masters and others have found that 50 percent of patients with angina had normal electrocardiograms; but when the patient's heart rate increases, the flow of blood should increase through the coronary arteries to the heart. If these coronary arteries are narrowed and not enough blood flows through them with an adequate oxygen supply, it is then that the patient experiences angina, and the electrocardiogram may display abnormalities not seen at rest.

The crude stress tests at that time consisted of jumping in place or running in place and then listening to the heart and recording an electrocardiogram. Dr. Masters devised a two-step test which resembles the stress test we are familiar with today. At the onset the patient went up and down a prescribed number of steps in set times (like thirty steps in three minutes). An electrocardiogram was taken at rest, and then when the patient had finished his two-step excursion, another electrocardiogram would be taken when his pulse was still high. Changes were then seen, chest pain was recorded, and the diagnosis of angina was confirmed or disproved.

It wasn't too long before a monitoring system came onto the scene. Electrodes were attached to the chest wall while the patient climbed up and down a series of steps and an electrocardiogram was recorded during his efforts. Soon, sophisticated exercise testing came into play, such as the bicycle and the treadmill.

The patient rides a bicycle or walks on a treadmill as his heart and blood pressure are monitored. If the patient develops chest pain while performing this procedure, the test is stopped and the electrocardiogram is studied for characteristic changes compatible with a positive test.

The major contention being debated throughout the medical community and the public arena is that stress tests are not of any value to a normal, healthy person, and that screening programs for such individuals are expensive and inconclusive. Glamorous statistical manipulations have indicated that, during a stress test, the reliability of a test is defined by the test sensitivity and specificity. The antistress cardiologists state, therefore, that it was unnecessary for President Carter to have a stress test before his jogging experience.

It is of no value to do stress tests on normal, healthy individuals who have no risk factors present, such as hypertension, smoking, family history of heart attack, and high cholesterol. Even persons engaged in hazardous occupations, like firemen and policemen, need not have a stress test if they are symptom free and have no risk factors.

We fully urge that a stress test be performed on asymptomatic patients over forty, whether they have a risk factor or not, if they plan to undertake any exercise program, especially vigorous exercise programs like jogging, tennis, racquetball, and others that require a large expenditure of energy. A recent newspaper item is included to illustrate its importance.

> DALLAS, March 14 (AP): Two crew members landed a Braniff International 747 jet safely today after they and two physicians were unable to revive the captain, who died at the controls en route from Honolulu to Dallas-Fort Worth.
>
> A Braniff spokesman, Jere Cox, said Capt. Lloyd Wilcox, 59 years old, of Dallas, apparently suffered a heart attack and became unconscious about 3 A.M. He had been a pilot for 35 years.
>
> Mr. Wilcox's wife, Terry, a flight attendant on the plane, told the authorities that her husband had complained of chest pains yesterday.
>
> James Cunningham, the co-pilot, and Robert Barnes, the second officer, landed the plane without incident at the Dallas-Fort Worth Airport at 6:19 A.M.
>
> Mr. Cox said the 331 passengers aboard Flight 502 were unaware of the captain's death. *New York Times,* March 15, 1979.

The purpose of the stress test is not only to determine if the patient has angina; many doctors fail to take into consideration that a stress test also identifies people who are at risk of sudden death. It is a well-known phenomenon that certain patients, although they are clinically asymptomatic and may not have coronary artery disease, develop irregular rhythms that are forerunners of the fatal rhythm of ventricular fibrillation. These prefatal arrhythmias sometimes can be identified with a properly conducted stress test. For example, some patients may develop an irregular rhythm and not be aware of it, their blood pressure may achieve dangerously high levels, and, in themselves, can bring on a heart attack or a stroke. Furthermore, some patients' cardiac reserves are so poor that the normal elevation of blood pressure and pulse that should follow exercise doesn't occur; the blood pressures may fall, and fainting episodes can result, and sometimes even sudden death.

It is true that many tests performed yield few positive results, and that from an economic point of view, the test may be unwarranted. However, as responsible physicians it is the individual with whom we are concerned, and whose life we need to save, even if it is one in a thousand. In the Talmud it is said that if you save one life, you save a generation. Stress testing can save lives. In a clinical setting it is indispensable in detailing when angina arrives and at what level, and in informing the patient how much he can do with reasonable safety. An exercise prescription cannot be written intelligently unless one knows at what level the patient reaches his physiological capacity without apparent danger.

Unfortunately, the abuse of the stress test is legion. Many nonphysicians are performing this test for profit. Health clubs, health clinics, spas, and rehabilitation centers, not run by physicians, are capitalizing on our medical knowledge. If and when a stress test is performed, it should be done only in the presence of a physician experienced in this procedure; otherwise it has little value. Stress testing is not the safest of all procedures: death can occur, as recorded in one in ten thousand patients studied.

There are patients who have severe triple-vessel disease who are totally asymptomatic when performing physical effort, but are prone to sudden death. Stress testing can identify these in at least two-thirds of the cases. As we have no means, other than cardiac catheterization, of identifying patients who are prone to die in this epidemic of coronary artery disease, we should use what we have, educate the public in its limitations, but not abandon it because statistics have shown invalidity in normal, healthy individuals.

Nearly forty years ago Dr. Arthur Masters recognized the stress test's limitations, never once was duped by a negative and positive finding, but relied on his great clinical experience. In the words of a famous surgeon, Dr. Claude Beck, "We must save hearts which are too young to die," and stress testing is an extra tool which the physician can use in this endeavor.

SPECIAL NOTE

CLASSIFICATIONS OF CARDIAC ILLNESS ACCORDING TO THE AMERICAN HEART ASSOCIATION

CARDIOLOGISTS AND SURGEONS like to classify cardiac illnesses into four groups:

Class I consists of patients who have heart disease, but ordinary physical activity does not cause them any discomfort.

Class II patients have cardiac disease with slight limitation of physical activity, but are quite comfortable at rest. Some activity results in fatigue, palpitations, and shortness of breath.

Class III are patients with cardiac disease resulting in marked limitation of physical activity. At rest, they are comfortable. Less than ordinary physical activity causes fatigue.

Class IV are patients with cardiac disease resulting in inability to carry on any physical activity at all without severe discomfort. Symptoms of cardiac failure are present even while the patient is at rest.

3: The Breast

Introduction

THE WOMAN sitting in a doctor's office has discovered a lump in her breast. After much hesitation she finally drummed up enough courage to seek help. She is afraid and anxious as all her thoughts race together: cancer, mutilation, family obligations, death—even before the biopsy is taken. The waiting is unbearable. She wants to know, swiftly, and dispense with all the formalities of insurance forms, past medical history, and so on. Biopsy it, remove it, cure it! Or is it too late for all that?

Such is the scene for hundreds of thousands of women each year; ninety-eight thousand of them have cancer and twenty-three thousand will die, but most lumps that women find in their breasts are not cancerous. Only 7 percent of women in the United States are afflicted, which means 93 percent never get cancer.

Lumps in the breast can occur at any age from fifteen to eighty years. The diagnosis, treatment, and choices involved in the final decision-making, in which women participate, will be discussed.

Function

For most of an adult woman's life, the breast is a nonsecreting, glandular structure encased in an envelope of fat. The breast, like the uterus, is affected by estrogen and undergoes cyclical changes. Prior to the onset of the monthly menses, the breasts are engorged because of the high production of ovarian estrogens. This engorgement accounts for the tenderness and irregular lumpiness of the breasts that women frequently experience during the premenstrual stage of the cycle. After ovulation and the reduction of ovarian estrogen, the breast engorgement subsides and so does the tenderness and lumpiness. The best time to have a breast examination is the fourteenth day after the onset of menses when the breasts are least tender and engorged.

Women at Risk to Have Cancer of the Breast

No one knows the cause of breast cancer. There are some historical traits that many cancer victims have in common. These women have fewer children and become pregnant at a later age than the national average. Cancer of the breast is more common among single women who have had no children. (For example, cancer of the breasts among nuns is higher than in the general population.) Breast cancer is said to run in families. There are numerous incidences in which a mother, daughter, sister, and even a grandparent develop the malignancy, or a mother, an aunt, and two daughters. One family, recorded by Dr. Brocca in 1866, had eight descendants—from a single grandmother—who developed cancer of the breast. Women with breast cancer transmit this predisposition or susceptibility to develop this cancer to their female offspring.

Women who have breast-fed their children seem to be more protected from cancer of the breast than women with a same number of pregnancies who have not breast-fed.

Cancers of the breast are, to some extent, stimulated by hormones, especially estrogen. In the laboratory this has been shown to be more evident in premenopausal women than postmenopausal women. Excessive production of estrogen due to ovarian imbalance or an ovarian growth is associated with high chances of developing breast cancer. The taking of estrogens is also believed by many to influence the occurrence of breast and uterine cancers. Other scientists disagree.

Women should take heart that cancer of the breast seems to have no relation to the amount of prolonged breast fondling or lovemaking. These questions are often asked, so we mention it now.

As the menstruating woman approaches menopause, the glandular elements of the breasts may be stimulated by unbalanced, aging ovaries which produce excessive estrogen. This sets the stage for excessive fibrous overgrowth and cystic dilation of the glands or of the ducts of the glands. Pathologists conclude that the development of fibrocystic changes occurs between the ages of thirty-five and fifty.

Age Determinants

The nature of the lump depends on the characteristic of the mass and the age of the patient.

AGE 16–25

Often a young woman will develop a tender mass prior to menses and be concerned about a lump. The "lump," on careful examination, turns out to be an underlying prominent rib, a diagnosis easily made by the experienced surgeon. Benign tumors can occur, but cancer of the breast in this age group is rare.

AGE 25–35

A mass discovered in such a patient is easily felt and has definite characteristics: smooth discrete margins, not attached to the underlying muscle or overlying skin of the breast; it is not tender and the other breast is normal.

This mass is benign and is called a fibroadenoma. As it is not malignant, it will not spread to other parts of the body. Surgeons confirm the diagnosis with X rays of the breasts (mammograms). This mass is better off removed, as it may increase in size. Cancer in this age bracket is rare.

AGE 40 PLUS

A lump found at this time of life can be a problem of diagnosis. An example will illustrate the dilemma.

A forty-eight-year-old woman had had a biopsy five years earlier which disclosed cysts of the breast. She is familiar with the swelling and tenderness that occurs in her breasts just before her periods. But this time the familiar ache shifted to the outer part of the breast and persisted. She thought she could feel a lump among the many irregularities in her breast. The examination of the breast displayed many irregularities and the most experienced examiner could not tell if there was a cancer among the clusters of cysts (fibrocystic disease of the breast).

Patients with fibrocystic disease may be at greater risk for the development of breast cancer. In this situation we would proceed with a mammography, needle aspiration of the cyst, and, possibly, biopsy.

Evaluation of the Patient with a Breast Mass (Mammograms)

Recently it has been reported that the best technique for the clinical evaluation of a lump in the breast is by repeated, properly conducted physical examinations. All the other techniques, such as mammography, are used to complement the experienced hand of the physician.

The breast examination should be performed in two positions: the patient lying down, and sitting up with hands on hips. In these positions the breasts can be effectively examined along with the armpits (axillary regions) and the hollows above the clavicles (collarbones). After the mass is confirmed, the next step is evaluation with mammography.

Mammography
(X-ray Examination of the Breast)

Mammography is useful for evaluating a mass in the breast. It has received unfavorable publicity because too many breast X rays were associated with increased incidence of cancer. Initially this procedure was used for screening thousands of women who showed no evidence of a mass in the physical examination. As the yield of early unsuspected cancers was small, the screening approaches have been abandoned.

The procedure is painless and is conducted in the privacy of an X-ray department. The X-ray technician places the breast on an X-ray plate and the cone of the machine is positioned above and alongside the breast. Two exposures, one from above and one from the side, are made of each breast. Interpretation of the mammogram is done by a radiologist. A mammogram has its limitations and can miss a cancerous lesion, especially if it develops behind a cyst.

An eighteen-year-old with tender premenstrual breasts should not have a mammogram. A forty-five-year-old woman known to have fibrocystic disease who develops a painful mass should undergo mammography. A postmenopausal woman who finds a lump in her breast should have a mammography to search for masses in the other breast.

RECOMMENDATIONS REGARDING MAMMOGRAPHY FROM THE NATIONAL INSTITUTES OF HEALTH

• Mammography and physical examination in combination should continue to be available on request to women fifty years of age or older. But there is no basis for such routine screening for women under the age of fifty. (This does not mean, however, that these women could not benefit from physical examination for breast cancer, and breast self-examination.)

• Mammography for women aged forty to forty-nine years should be restricted to women having a personal history of breast cancer, or whose mothers or sisters have a history of breast cancer.

• Mammographic screening of women aged thirty-five to thirty-nine years should be limited to those women having a personal history of breast cancer.

• There are no rigorous scientific data to show to what extent either physical examination alone or mammography alone is beneficial.

• Mammographic techniques have improved markedly in recent years with smaller, and presumably earlier, lesions now being detected; moreover, radiation dosage has been decreased significantly. Nonetheless, there are no data to indicate that these advances result in decreased mortality in women under age fifty.

Fibrocystic Disease of the Breast (Cysts of the Breast)

Evaluating the woman with advanced fibrocystic disease is a difficult problem for the surgeon. Fear that a cancer may be dwelling among the numerous cysts is a constant concern. Along with mammographic examinations, the surgeon may perform needle aspiration of the lump. If fluid can be successfully aspirated from the mass and it disappears completely, no further treatment is necessary, except repeated careful follow-up examinations. If the mass cannot be aspirated, or if after it is aspirated it does not disappear completely, then a biopsy is performed.

Technique of Needle Aspiration of a Cyst

This procedure can be performed in the office with or without local anesthesia. A needle is inserted through the skin into the cyst after the skin has been cleansed with an antiseptic. The fluid is then aspirated into the syringe and can be sent to the laboratory to be examined under the microscope for cells. Most of the time the cell examination is not helpful. The breast is examined after aspiration and again four to six weeks thereafter. Reappearance of the mass requires biopsy.

Breast Biopsy for Suspicious Mass

When the mammographic finding reveals changes compatible with a malignancy, further noninvasive testing is abandoned and tissue is obtained for microscopic examination. The patient is admitted to the hospital and undergoes a series of tests that search for spread of cancer to the lungs, liver, and bones. These tests are called liver scans and bone scans and are included along with blood tests and chest X ray.

Traditionally, the patient is prepared for the breast biopsy to be followed immediately by the mastectomy if the pathologist confirms that the biopsy reveals cancer. After almost seventy years this arrangement has been challenged and alternatives will be discussed later in the chapter.

Description of the Biopsy and Surgery

The night before, shaving of the breast area is done in the event that a mastectomy is required, and a sleeping pill is given.

The operating theater for breast cancer is very special. As, today, many of the staff are women, they feel personally involved in each operation, almost as if their own breasts are about to be explored. The entire room is filled with great anxiety and prayer that the lesion is not cancerous.

In recent years the timing as well as the technique of the breast biopsy has received considerable attention and publicity. Many surgeons and women's groups are now suggesting that a biopsy, when technically possible, be carried out in the surgeon's office or outpatient clinic prior to hospitalization, along with screening blood work and even the bone scan. One technique, called needle biopsy, is performed by injecting a small amount of local anesthetic in the region of the tumor and inserting a special needle designed to obtain a small specimen. The surgeon, in the office, may elect to make a small incision in the area to obtain a portion of the mass for microscopic examination before the patient is hospitalized.

Prior to mastectomy, if the mass does prove to be malignant, a full discussion of the surgical treatment can be carried out with the patient and her family. The diagnosis and possible mastectomy are separated from each other by two to three days, allowing the woman to decide, with the advice of her surgeon, whether a partial or complete mastectomy should be performed, or radiation therapy.

Although many surgeons claim that this is better psychological preparation, it has been the authors' experience that many patients prefer to be managed in the more traditional fashion. This is particularly true when they have known the surgeon for some time and have confidence in his or her judgment. They would rather have the biopsy and the surgery performed at one time and oppose the crusade for "two-step surgery." We believe a compromise is possible. After thorough discussion and examination, it is the woman who will decide whether she wishes the traditional one-step operation or the two-stage procedure.

If the mass has been identified microscopically as a malignancy, surgical removal of any possible residual tumor along with an adequate margin of normal tissue is now required. The best surgical procedure to accomplish this end has become a matter of considerable controversy. Most surgeons, with the agreement of internists specializing in chemotherapy (oncologists), have abandoned the previously time-honored radical mastectomy.

This procedure, described by William Halsted eighty-five years ago, remained the choice of operation until recently. A radical mastectomy means the complete removal of the involved breast, the underlying two muscles from the front of the chest, and a thorough cleaning of the contents of the axilla (armpit) on that side of the chest. Today the lesser procedures give equal curative and palliative results and the radical operation is no longer popular.

Once there is the slightest evidence that a tumor has spread beyond the confines of the breast, such as to the axillary nodes, it is presumed that the disease is widespread. Surgery limited to the area of the involved breast and the corresponding axillary region is not sufficient, and chemotherapy, called *adjuvant therapy*, is added.

The twelve to fifty lymph nodes in the axillary area can become involved by the cancer in the breast through drainage ducts, called *lymphatic vessels*, that lead from the breast to the armpit. It is crucial to determine the number of lymph nodes involved, the greater the number, the more widespread the cancer and the worse the prognosis. This is true even if there is no X-ray or laboratory evidence of such spread. If lymph nodes are involved, survival after five years is 50 to 60 percent. In two to eight years there may be spread to the bones, lungs, brain, liver, or other organs.

Staging or Degree of Progression of the Cancer

Cancers of the breast are classified according to the stage or degree of progression of the disease at the time of the diagnosis and from the tissue removed at surgery. The type of operative procedure depends on the degree of progression of the disease as determined by physical examination, laboratory data, and scans to determine spread of the disease to other organs. The prognosis of the patient is statistically correlated with the extent or stage of the cancer.

Stage I cancers have the best prognosis, the tumor size being no larger than 2 cm in diameter. They are freely movable (they are not attached to the overlying skin of the breast, nor to the underlying muscle of the chest wall). Examination of the armpit on the same side reveals no lymph node enlargement. Patients with stage I cancer of the breast have a greater than 80 percent chance of ten-year survival.

Stage II lesions are 2 cm to 5 cm in diameter and the axilla may have enlarged lymph nodes. Generally these masses are not fixed to the underlying muscle or other overlying skin. Then ten-year survival is approximately 60 percent and these patients generally will receive chemotherapy following mastectomy.

Stage III cancers of the breast are greater than 5 cm in diameter and the cancer clearly extends to the skin of the breast or is fixed to the underlying chest muscles. Usually the lymph nodes in the armpit are infiltrated with cancer. The ten-year survival from this type is less than 30 percent. Following mastectomy these patients are recommended to have adjuvant chemotherapy.

Stage IV cancer of the breast indicates the cancer to have grown beyond the breast into the axilla, resulting in fixation of the axillary nodes, or there may be complete fixation of the tumor to the chest wall and evidence of spread to distant regions, such as bone, brain, or lungs. The chance of surviving five years with stage IV cancer of the breast is in the area of 10 percent.

Historical Review

In 1894 a brilliant surgeon in Baltimore, Maryland, by the name of Halsted, developed a radical mastectomy. In the late 1800s and the early part of this century women did not come to the doctor early for their cancers but waited until there was a huge ulcer or such a large mass that they could no longer ignore it or even live with it.

The operation to remove it, therefore, had to be extensive and radical. Because of the size of the cancers, the condition of the patients, and medical knowledge at that time, up to 23 percent of women undergoing such surgery died while in the hospital. Surgeons reported the chances of surviving three years from the time of diagnosis was somewhere between 5 to 30 percent. As a result of Halsted's brilliant work survival rates increased and mortality rates from the operation decreased. In 1907 Halsted reported that close to 35 percent of women survived three years and almost 30 percent survived five years following the diagnosis. He reduced the chances of dying from the operation to less than 3 percent. Halsted's operation described removal of the major muscle of the front of the chest along with cleaning out the lymph glands from the axilla. Modifications of this work were described as early as 1906 and again in 1938. However, it was not until recent times that the radical mastectomy was largely abandoned and more conservative procedures were championed by surgeons throughout the world.

Contemporary Surgery

For stage I or selected stage II breast cancers most surgeons now recommend total removal of the breast and a significant cleanout of the axillary lymph glands so that twelve to fifteen of them can be studied microscopically. Considerable argument and controversy throughout the medical world exists about stage I or selected stage II cancers.

Some surgeons champion a much more conservative approach. A partial, or *hemi-mastectomy,* is now performed by increasing numbers of surgeons for these very selected cases, along with a cleanout or dissection of the axilla. The dissection of the axilla may have to be done through a separate second incision. It has been pointed out by a small group of surgeons that such a limited removal of breast tissue should be followed by radiation treatment after healing of the surgical incision. This is not the current practice in the United States.

Most stage II and all stage III cancers should be treated with total mastectomy and thorough axillary cleanout. This is generally referred to as an *extended mastectomy,* or a *modified radical mastectomy.* Some surgeons, when performing a modified radical mastectomy, additionally remove a minor muscle from the chest wall. The incision for a modified radical mastectomy, or extended simple mastectomy, is usually traverse so that the incision cannot be seen above a standard brassiere or low-cut dress, or even in a bathing suit. Occasionally, when the cancer is a large, bulky mass that ulcerates the skin and has been neglected, immediate surgery may not be possible. Pre-operative radiation therapy to shrink the tumor may initially be advisable followed by removal of the breast.

Recently a patient came to our office with a small tumor in the left breast with some redness of the skin. She had been limping for three weeks and complained of pain in the right hip. X rays and bone scan showed destruction of bone in the hip from cancerous spread. This woman did not have a mastectomy, but was treated with radiation and chemotherapy. The hip pain is now gone and the breast mass has shrunk. Although she is doing well, the chance of her surviving five years is not greater than 10 percent.

Radiation

In years past, radiation therapy was an intrinsic part of the treatment of cancer of the breast. Stage II or III lesions were radiated to destroy residual cancer cells in the mastectomy site, in the area of the axilla, and above the clavicle along the area of the breastbone or sternum. After many years it was realized that the combination of radical mastectomy and radiation therapy did not protect the patient from recurrences in more distant areas, such as the brain, lungs, and bones. It became clear that the treatment was adequate only for the local area of the breast. Recurrences after five years, at distant sites, made it evident that there were dormant cells that had already spread prior to the mastectomy and were not destroyed by the radiation treatment.

The Best Survival Occurs with Earlier Diagnosis

The tumor of smaller size with no spread (metastasis) is associated with longer survival rates. Yet, in spite of these facts, most women are hesitant to examine themselves regularly to find breast masses. Unfortunately, even today, there are women who, on finding a mass, will not visit a doctor, for they fear being told they have cancer, they fear the treatments, and they fear the loss of a breast.

In most cases, breast cancer is not a local disease and, hence, local treatment will not suffice, but treatment called *systemic therapy*, involving the entire body, is used. Systemic therapy can either take the form of chemotherapy, hormonal manipulation, and even perhaps a new treatment called immunotherapy, used to prolong life and provide cures.

All cancers are fickle and unpredictable. Their growth rate and time of spread may vary from individual to individual.

Hormonal Treatment

Recent findings indicate a way to distinguish two types of breast cancers, which may have very different prognoses. In one group of women, breast tumors depend upon hormones for growth; whereas in the other, the malignancy continues to multiply independent of the hormone stimulation. The group of women whose breast tumors are positive for estrogen receptors have a much lower rate of recurrence after mastectomy, if they recur at all, than do patients whose tumors are not estrogen dependent.

In every modern hospital in the United States a portion of the cancer in the breast is sent to the laboratory to be tested for these hormone receptors, the breast being sensitive to cyclic hormone changes taking place in a woman's body. Some of these tumors are found to have receptors to estrogen or to progesterone, or to both. Even patients whose cancer has spread to the lymph nodes have a better prognosis if their estrogen receptors are positive. In the presence of metastases of the breast to the various organs, such as bone, brain, lung, and so forth, it has been demonstrated that 40 to 60 percent of patients with positive estrogen receptors, when treated with hormonal manipulation, will show objective evidence of tumor regression.

In the past when metastases were found in premenopausal women, it was traditional to remove the ovaries and other endocrine organs to eliminate the source of estrogen. The first attempt was performed by a surgeon, George Beston, of Glasgow, in 1895, who removed the ovaries of two afflicted women. Thus was born the hormonal therapy of breast cancer, antedating radiation and chemotherapy. Several controlled trials, including the National Surgical Adjuvant and Breast Project, disclosed that removal of the ovaries by surgery or by radiation and/or the use of hormones that oppose estrogens causes a significant remission in spread of the cancer and prolongs the tumor-free period or the period before recurrence.

Medical treatment of breast cancer must be administered by physicians who specialize in oncology. This relatively new specialty has made an enormous impact on all forms of cancers, especially on cancer of the breast. Today a surgeon is remiss if he does not involve an oncologist as part of the team, along with the family physician.

Hormonal therapy is combined more often than not with chemotherapy. Surgeons and oncologists agree that hormonal therapy and chemotherapy are useful and indispensable in the treatment of stages II through V. The patient with a stage II or III cancer must be protected against recurrence of her illness from dormant cells that have already spread to the bone or the brain. Even if partial or complete mastectomy is done, adjuvant chemotherapy must also be employed. This method kills or retards the growth of cancer cells by the administration of medications either by injection or orally.

Chemotherapy

In 1934 Liston Dustin discovered, almost by accident, that colchicine, a drug that is four thousand years old and used in the treatment of gout, also blocks the division of normal cells. In 1940 Dr. S. A. Waxman, who received the Nobel prize for the discovery of streptomycin, also discovered actinomycin, derived from mushrooms, which had anticancer properties.

Discoveries and cures often result from keen observations during accidents or crises. A notable example was demonstrated when, in 1943, the Liberty ship *John E. Harvey*, torpedoed in the North Sea, sank with one hundred tons of mustard gas aboard. A bright young naval doctor by the name of Peter Alexander observed that the white count of survivors was markedly diminished. Alert laboratory researchers took note of this report and began to experiment with this drug's effect on dividing blood and tumor cells. Mustard gas was tried in 1946 as an anticancer agent and it was the first class of anticancer drugs called *alkylating agents*.

At the present time there are dozens upon dozens of medications being tested and used for chemotherapy of the breast. Single drugs or combinations are used, but all forms of treatment may have some complications. Some are minor, such as hair loss; more serious, and sometimes fatal, complications are overwhelming infections and heart disease. All in all, patients tolerate the medications with ease and are gratified by their results.

Adjuvant therapy, or chemotherapy, given at the time of mastectomy, evolved from observations made by Bernard Fischer on the recurrence rate of breast cancer. He discovered that patients with no positive axillary nodes at the time of surgery have a local and distant recurrence rate of 20 percent at five years, and 24 percent at ten years; with one to three positive nodes, recurrence rates are 53 percent and 65 percent at five and ten years; with four or more nodes, there is an 80 percent chance of recurrence at five years and 86 percent at ten years. Once recurrence has occurred in breast cancer, patients will eventually succumb to their illness.

At the present time studies are being performed to determine if adjuvant therapy is of any use in patients with negative axillary nodes at the time of surgery. Even today, therapy changes so swiftly that it is not possible to suggest guidelines.

Patients should take heart that an enormous amount of research and trials is being performed with different drug combinations with gratifying results. As Dr. Joseph Bertino, of the Yale University Medical School, stated, "Not so long ago, chemotherapy was considered a last resort for breast cancer patients. Now we know that some cancers respond exceedingly well to treatment with a combination of drugs and we may use chemotherapy as a first rather than a last method."

Other Points of View

The entire approach to the treatment and diagnosis of cancer of the breast is in constant change. For example, ten years ago only 13 percent of patients were treated with the modified mastectomy. Five years ago this went up to 23 percent, and in 1977 the figure had climbed to 44 percent, and it appears that the radical Halsted operation is being totally abandoned.

Operations are now being performed which are even less extensive than the modified radical mastectomy. For example, Dr. Maurice S. Fox published a paper in 1979 examining the results of surgery done in Britain, Denmark, and the United States in which only the cancerous lump plus the surrounding tissues were removed from the woman's breast, followed by intense radiation therapy. The ten-year survival rates of women treated with radical mastectomy and those treated with *lumpectomy,* or a simple segmental therapy plus radiation, were exactly the same.

Other proponents of the relatively minimal surgery plus aggressive radiation are Ira Goldenberg, Professor of Surgery at Yale Medical School, and Oliver Cope, Professor of Surgery at Harvard. For two decades Dr. Cope has treated hundreds of patients with breast cancer and is convinced that standard surgical procedures cured only those patients whose cancers are confined to the breast: 25 percent of all women with breast malignancy. The other 75 percent are women whose cancers already had spread to other parts of the body through the lymph nodes or the bloodstream. In women with strictly localized cancers, a small operation would be sufficient, Dr. Cope noted. Deaths from cancer of the breast result from spread rather than local recurrences.

Dr. Ira Goldenberg states: "Radiation technology has improved enormously during the past five years. We have used radiation on inoperable cancers for a long time. Now, with our ability to concentrate more powerful X-rays on localized areas, we know that we can destroy cancers as effectively with radiation as with surgery. The accessibility of the breast makes it relatively easy to deliver curative dosage with minimal damage to underlying tissues. Local excision plus radiation will, of course, leave the breast with a scar plus some shrinking and discoloration. Cosmetically, this damage is almost invisible when the woman is clothed."

These physicians advocate a simple surgical operation consisting of removal of the tumor, with or without some of the lymph nodes, leaving the breast in place, followed by radiation.

Recent well-publicized studies have described an 80 percent relapse rate of five years for patients with four or more axillary nodes involved by cancer at the time of mastectomy and a 50 percent relapse rate of patients with one to three nodes involved. Adjuvant chemotherapy has been advocated because the disease relapse rates are so high and chemotherapy cures are not obtainable at present after overt metastatic disease appears. Because of these disheartening statistics, trials are now being performed to try to use adjuvant therapy at the time of surgery.

Drs. Cope and Goldenberg's views are still highly controversial within the medical community, and not the standard form of treatment. At the Sixth Annual Breast Cancer Symposium, sponsored by a number of top cancer research centers and held in New York in January 1979, most of the panel members still talked in terms of mastectomy as opposed to lumpectomy as the treatment of choice. Lumpectomy followed by radiation is not considered the current form of treatment and is not advised by the majority of surgeons. Lumpectomy and removal of axillary nodes, not followed by radiation, is closer to what surgeons will accept.

Follow-up Care after Mastectomy

All patients must have careful follow-up treatment after mastectomy. Patients who are stage I should be seen initially every three months for three years and thereafter at least every six months. Stage II and III patients similarly must be seen by the surgeon every three months; this should be continued for five years. Stage II and III patients, of course, should be meeting regularly with the oncologist for therapy. In all of these patients repeated laboratory evaluation searching for evidence of metastatic disease to liver, bone, or lungs is indicated.

A new test called CEA (carcinoembryonic antigen) is based on an antigen produced by the body in the presence of a malignancy, such as one originating in the breast. It may be that this antigen becomes positive before any other tests do, indicating that the tumor has recurred. Consequently many surgeons and internists order this test routinely at regular intervals. If the finding should suddenly change from a normal to an abnormal range, further investigation is indicated. As an early indicator of otherwise clinically undetectable appearances, this test is still controversial, however.

Breast Reconstruction after Mastectomy

Dressing and undressing for some patients becomes a daily nightmare, reminding them of their cancer operation. In some cases the marriage suffers and sexual relations cease. For some women the answer has been breast reconstruction. This is a relatively new approach to the cosmetic problems following a mastectomy and the indications and restrictions of the procedure are now changing.

Ideally, breast reconstruction is limited to women with stage I disease who have had a complete mastectomy. Women with stage II and sometimes stage III disease have also demanded breast reconstruction and have had the procedure successfully carried out.

Since radical mastectomy has been largely abandoned for more conservative operations, the muscles of the chest wall are left in place. This makes reconstruction of the breast relatively straightforward. A so-called bag is implanted in a pocket beneath the main muscle of the chest, forming a contour and mound of the breast. The nipple can be reconstructed from a portion of the nipple on the opposite breast, or even from donor tissue in the vaginal region.

In the authors' experience, the number of patients undergoing this procedure has been small, but the interest is clearly growing and the operation will undoubtedly be requested by more women.

Cancer of the Breast in Men

Cancer in the male breast represents less than 1 percent of all the breast cancers seen in the United States. Usually cancer appears as a painless firm nodule beneath and attached to the nipple. The diagnosis is usually made late, when there is involvement of the axillary lymph nodes.

Unilateral or bilateral swelling of the male breast around the nipple area, called *gynecomastia,* can occur as a result of certain medications, such as digitalis, for example, and in medical conditions, such as cirrhosis of the liver. Likewise, gynecomastia can occur in the male receiving female hormones for cancer of the prostate. If no biopsy is recommended, a second opinion is indicated. Neglected cancer of the male breast is a lethal disease, but early diagnosis can be lifesaving.

Treatment is usually mastectomy with the removal of some of the chest wall muscles. If the diagnosis has been made early and the axillary lymph nodes are free of cancer, there is an 80 percent chance of five-year survival. If the axillary lymph nodes are involved in the cancer, the chance of survival for five years is reduced to about 25 percent. Male patients with cancer of the breast seem to respond to hormonal treatment, which results in some regression of the malignancy for a period of time.

4: Hysterectomy

TOO LONG HAS THE WOMAN STOOD BY as an outsider, allowing her body to be surgically violated for the removal of female organs. Now is the time for her to participate in the decision-making. This is only possible through more education and understanding of the alternatives available. Most women are learning something about themselves from reading current popular magazines or from talk shows and women's organizations. Bits of information (many times false) trickle down at them from neighbors, mothers-in-law, and friends. Old wives' tales, rumors, and health magazines perplex them, leaving them confused and frightened concerning hysterectomy.

Hysterectomy is the second most frequent major operation performed today. We are living in a time when nearly half of all women in the United States are advised at some time to have a hysterectomy. More than 800,000 women had hysterectomies in 1979, paying approximately $500 million in fees.

A congressional committee estimated that 25 percent of hysterectomies are either unjustified or unnecessary. In his book,

Dr. Lawrence P. Williams stated that "hysterectomy ranks second after tonsillectomies in the number of unnecessary operations performed yearly." The *Ladies' Home Journal* also published an article entitled "Needless Hysterectomy" in March of 1976. These articles, along with government support of the notion of second opinion and urging of insurance carriers to pay for this opinion, leave a woman with an enormous dilemma. The obstetrician who has carried her through her deliveries has now become her gynecologist. Must she look at him with a jaundiced eye if he recommends hysterectomy?

We plan to present preeminent U.S. gynecologists' opinions regarding hysterectomies. Ample explanations are included to assist you in making educated decisions and choices. Some of these opinions may differ among gynecologists, but this is how it is practiced in our medical community.

The Major Indications for Hysterectomy in the United States

Out of the 800,000 hysterectomies performed each year, 30 percent are due to myomas of the uterus, also known as fibroid tumors; cancers, 15 percent; prolapse operations, 35 percent; and sterilization, 20 percent. Two-thirds of the operations are done by an abdominal incision and one-third vaginally. The overall mortality rate has been estimated to be approximately one thousand women per year.

The Approaches for Removal of the Uterus

In an abdominal hysterectomy the removal of the uterus is accomplished through an abdominal incision. The incision may be a vertical or a horizontal one, called the bikini incision. In a *vaginal hysterectomy* an incision is made on the vagina through which the uterus is removed.

The type of surgery to be performed depends on the illness. For instance, when a hysterectomy is done for large fibroids and certain types of cancer, the operation is usually done by the abdominal method. Other times, the vaginal or the abdominal method may be used, depending on the surgeon's recommendations.

Vaginal hysterectomies are sometimes the only method used, as when there is prolapse of the uterus associated with conditions that will be discussed briefly, such as cystoceles, rectoceles, and enteroceles.

A vaginal hysterectomy has the following advantages: 1) absence of scar; 2) shorter hospital stay; 3) little pain and discomfort; 4) fewer complications; 5) shorter recovery period; and 6) a shorter operation with the patient under anesthesia for less time. The major disadvantage of the vaginal hysterectomy is that ovaries and tubes cannot be removed.

The advantages of the abdominal hysterectomy are: 1) the surgeon will be able to do a complete examination of the abdomen for pathology that he may not have expected; 2) the removal of the ovaries if necessary and the appendix if the patient so desires can be done; and 3) there is reportedly less infection in the postoperative period. The major disadvantage is that recovery time is longer, usually two to four weeks, a scar is visible, and complication rates may be higher. Sometimes the ovaries can also be removed during a vaginal hysterectomy.

Historical Aspects

The first gynecologist probably was the Egyptian goddess Tefnut, who prescribed milk and semen and berries of the poppy plant to produce milk in the breasts of women. Likewise, Hippocrates was an excellent gynecologist who wrote about menstruation, pregnancy, and lactation.

For centuries women have been the victims of bizarre practices. For example, wild cucumber pulp in breast milk would promote menstruation and lion's fat softened by rose oil would aid conception. Egyptian papyrus records advise "tips of aci mixed with honey and applied to a piece of lint which is placed in the vagina," or, to accelerate the birth of a child, "pepper-mint leaves—apply it to her bare posterior." For a girl's breasts, "nine pellets of hair dug into the liquid" were uplifting. And to allay offensive odors from armpits, "apply blood from a lamb's amputated testicles." Ashes of a burned lizard wrapped in linen were aphrodisiacs when held in the left hand, or eating the eye of a hyena with licorice and dill would cause a woman to conceive, and this was guaranteed within three days. And so it went.

It was in the nineteenth century that gynecology became a separate specialty. The first modern hysterectomy was performed on a patient by the name of Jane Todd Crawford, who, at the age of forty-seven, thought herself to be pregnant. The year was 1809 and a doctor named Effren McDowell who lived sixty miles away was sent for. It was he who is credited with performing the first hysterectomy. Jane Crawford was taken by horseback on a sixty-mile journey to the town of Danville, Kentucky, where the operation was performed; she lived to the age of seventy-eight. The surgery performed by this frontier physician was to remove a huge ovarian tumor, without the benefit of general anesthesia and sterile technique. He did use mixtures of opium to dull the pain. By 1840 surgery was well on its way but the mortality rate was so high from infections that few women consented to be operated on.

Pregnancy was marked by severe infections, called puerperal fever, and frequent deaths until the brilliant physician Ignaz Semmelweis from Budapest made the astute observation that medical students and professors left the dissecting room after postmortem examinations carrying contaminated cadaveric material into the labor room and the lying-in wards, where the women became infected, developed fever, and died.

In 1847 Semmelweis revolutionized the practice of obstetrics and gynecology by instructing all his students to scrub their hands in a solution of chloride of lime before they delivered, examined, or touched any patient. The death rate in the wards fell from 11 percent to 3 percent in one year. The medical profession and the press made a mockery out of this observation. Cartoons and obscene drawings depicted Semmelweis' new method. The practice of washing hands before deliveries was used by the Egyptians and the Greeks, but thousands of years had to pass before the woman again received adequate protection from infection.

Anatomy of the Female Reproductive System

The first formal description of the uterus was written by Soranus, who practiced in Rome during the time of Hadrian in the year A.D. 98. This is only a small part of his voluminous description:

> The uterus is situated in the space between the hip joints and between the bladder and the rectum, resting on a ladder and beneath the bladder, sometimes wholly and sometimes partly, because of changing its position according to its size. In children, the womb is smaller than the bladder, wherefore it is likely that it is entirely under the bladder, but in virgins at puberty it is equal to the bladder in height.

The female reproductive system is composed of the vulva, the vagina, the uterus, the tubes, and the ovaries. The vulva consists of the labia, which are two raised folds of tissue covering the clitoris—a small erectile organ—and the urinary opening through which urine is passed. The vagina and its canal lie below the meatus and above the rectum. On either side of the vagina are two small glands which secrete mucus for lubrication. The vaginal canal leads to the uterus. The lower portion of the uterus that extends into the vagina is the cervix. Above the cervix is the body of the uterus, a small organ extending from which are the fallopian tubes.

The Physiology of the Reproductive System

Estrogens and progesterones, hormones produced from the ovaries and other glands, are responsible for breast growth and development of sexual organs. Production of these hormones decreases between the ages of 45 and 55, and, when menstruation ceases, menopause begins.

The ovaries, attached to the back of the uterus, produce one mature egg each month, and this is called ovulation. Toward the middle of a menstrual cycle the mature egg escapes, and the hormones secreted from the ovaries prepare the uterus for conception.

The Diagnostic Examination

A thorough obstetrical and gynecological history is taken by the examining physician, and a family history is mandatory. The surgeon must identify women with family histories of cancer to help in the decision on whether to advise surgery.

A pelvic examination is then performed to estimate the size and position of the uterus and to determine the presence of tumors as well as abnormalities of the ovaries.

The cervix is visualized through a speculum and observations are made on the presence of erosions, atrophy, and discolorations. A smear of the cells is taken—a pap smear—for microscopic study to detect cancer of the cervix. A pap smear that is suspicious must be repeated. If it is positive for cancer, a biopsy of the cervix is taken.

ULTRASONOGRAPHY

We have seen the use of ultrasonography, or echocardiography, in studying the heart. It is also useful in identifying ovarian cysts, fibroid tumors, and pregnancy in the tubes or in the uterus.

ENDOMETRIAL BIOPSY

A small hollow probe is introduced through the vagina and into the uterus and a piece of tissue removed for microscopic examination.

DILATATION AND CURETTAGE

Commonly known by the acronym D & C, this is by far the most common gynecological procedure. It is both diagnostic and therapeutic and can be performed in the physician's office or as a surgical procedure under anesthesia in the hospital. This procedure is used for diagnosis to obtain biopsy specimens from a variety of areas which then can be given to the pathologist to study. It can be therapeutic when performed to treat a bleeding problem or to remove the contents of the uterus, as in the case of an incomplete or therapeutic abortion. Under local or general anesthesia, the cervix is dilated and an instrument with a spoonlike curette is used to scrape the lining of the uterus.

Myths Regarding Hysterectomies

Old wives' tales and misinformation have afflicted the woman with needless concerns about the aftermath of hysterectomies. Some women fear that it will not be possible to have sexual enjoyments after a hysterectomy and that they will lose their "womanhood." It is the same type of fear men have when the prostate is removed. The uterus is not a sexual organ, per se, and has little to do with enjoyment of sex. Other myths suggest that women will age faster, gain weight, their skin will look old and wrinkled, and hair growth will increase. Other unjustified misunderstandings are the onset of depression, forgetfulness, and insanity.

In spite of the bad propaganda, most women experience few, if any, major problems following a hysterectomy. Later on in the chapter some of the complications that may arise and that are not myths will be discussed.

Timing of the Operation

There are occasions when the uterus must be removed with either one or both tubes and ovaries in an emergency situation in order to save the life of a patient, as when the pregnancy is located outside the uterus, usually in the fallopian tubes. In most instances a hysterectomy is not an emergency procedure; it is then classified as either the elective procedure or the non-elective procedure.

NONELECTIVE PROCEDURE

This type of operation is performed to save the patient's life if or when it is a constant threat to her well-being; for example, patients who have continued bleeding—women who cease to take the oral contraceptive pill for whatever reasons may have heavy, uncontrolled bleeding, requiring hysterectomy—or patients with a large uterus with benign tumors (noncancerous) that interfere with the function of other organs.

ELECTIVE PROCEDURE

These are performed for conditions that are not threatening and do not impair general health but interfere with the comfort of the patient, for example, prolapse of the uterus, or when the uterus slips out of place. Although sterilization procedures by performing hysterectomy are not common in today's society, some patients and surgeons still decide to accomplish sterilization by removing the uterus.

Other operations that are performed in association with a hysterectomy consist of 1) a cystocele, which is a rupture or herniation of the bladder into the vagina; 2) the repair of a rectocele, a herniation of the rectal wall into the vagina; 3) repair of an enterocele, a herniation of the intestine into the vagina between the wall of the rectum and cervix.

Complications of Hysterectomies

Complications may be major or minor, and most of the time are rare. Complications will be lessened depending on the general condition of the patient before the operation, the skill of the surgeon, and the facility in which the patient is operated on. Some complications are not unique to hysterectomies but are common to most operations and are briefly mentioned below.

EXCESSIVE BLEEDING

When the surgeon operates under conditions in which many blood vessels need to be severed, excessive bleeding may result. Blood transfusion is then indicated.

INFECTIONS

Major infections are rare, minor infections common, especially if the operation is done through the vagina. More serious infections may localize in the pelvic cavity, giving rise to an infection of the lining of the abdomen, called *peritonitis.* This may occur anywhere after four to six weeks. Today, with excellent antibiotics available, infections, as a rule, are readily controlled and eliminated. The surgeon will have no hesitancy in asking a second opinion from an infectious disease expert if the infection appears to be poorly controlled.

FISTULA WITH LOSS OF URINE

This is a rare complication that results when an abnormal opening develops between the urinary bladder, the ureters, and the tubes that carry the urine from the kidneys to the bladder and the vagina. This generally occurs in patients who have been treated previously with radium and in cancer patients; it can also be inadvertently caused by the surgeon. In this condition the patient loses urine through the vagina and corrective surgery is generally performed to mend this situation. A similar fistula, an opening between the intestine and the vagina, may occur, with a loss of feces through the vagina— another rare complication that the surgeon will correct.

PHLEBITIS

Pelvic surgery lends itself to phlebitis, especially when cancer operations are performed. Patients who are predisposed to this complication are generally those who are obese or have been on birth control pills. When a clot forms in the veins and travels to the lungs, we speak of pulmonary embolism, which, unfortunately, sometimes is associated with sudden death several days after surgery. Most surgeons employ precautions to avoid this complication by using a medication which prevents clots, called heparin.

PULMONARY COMPLICATIONS

Occasionally, postoperatively, patients can develop pneumonia and partial collapse of the lung, or *atelectasis*. This condition is more likely to occur in patients who are heavy smokers or in obese women. The cough reflex may be suppressed by their receiving too many medications to control pain, and the general lassitude of the breathing mechanism is a proper setting for infections. To avoid this complication, the surgeon and nursing staff will urge the patient to breathe deeply and cough frequently, and to use instruments to clear the lungs, such as blowing up a balloon or a positive pressure respiratory device.

SUMMARY

The better the condition of the patient prior to surgery, the more likely the patient is going to heal with fewer complications. Patients who are obese or are heavy smokers, or who have other associated diseases, such as diabetes and lung disease, will have more complications.

Many of the complications cited for hysterectomy are common to many of the other surgical procedures, especially if general anesthesia is used.

FIBROID TUMORS, OR MYOMAS

It is estimated that nearly 40 percent of women at the age of fifty have fibroids, and, for some unknown reason, black women are more likely to have fibroids than white women. This is the most common nonmalignant disease of the uterus.

A fibroid is a benign tumor consisting of the same muscle as the uterus, varying in size from a pea to a watermelon. Sometimes it becomes so large that it fills the entire abdominal cavity like a pregnant uterus. More than one fibroid may be present.

Symptoms

A fibroid tumor may be totally asymptomatic, found during a checkup, or it may cause the patient undue abnormal bleeding and pressure symptoms. If the tumor is large, it may push on the bladder or rectum, causing inability to hold the urine. If fibroids are very large and located on the side of the uterus, they sometimes obstruct the ureters and cause kidney troubles. When the fibroid is on a stalk, it might twist and cause severe recurrent pain.

When to Operate on a Myoma of the Uterus

As fibroid tumors are present in four out of every ten women between the ages of forty and fifty, most gynecologists feel removal is indicated when it gives rise to repeated abnormal bleeding during menstruation and between periods. The bleeding can be so heavy, resulting in loss of blood, that it makes the patient chronically weak. When a gynecologist first finds a myoma and it begins to grow rapidly, this is also a strong indication for removal along with a hysterectomy. Rarely, rapid growth suggests a malignant change in the myoma.

When the myoma is the size of a twelve-week pregnancy, or grapefruit size, most gynecologists contemplate an operation.

When Not to Operate

If the surgeon advises an operation for a fibroid tumor that, on the first visit, is not at least the size of a grapefruit, a second opinion is warranted. If the myoma is asymptomatic and is not of the size mentioned before, the gynecologist must determine how long it has been there, how rapidly it has been growing, and to what extent it impinges upon adjacent organs. Back pain may be caused by myoma, but is not an indication to perform surgery unless other causes of back pain are ruled out.

Fibroids depend on hormones for growth and most regress after the menopause. Finding an asymptomatic myoma is not an indication for its removal or hysterectomy. If the general condition of the patient is poor and there are associated medical problems, such as a severe heart or lung disease, operations should not be performed. As menopause is approached, the fibroid should not be operated on unless there is an increase in size or suspicion of cancer. A myoma that causes uterine bleeding should not be operated on unless a D & C has been tried to control the bleeding, as this will help 80 percent of the time. Sometimes the fibroid is removed without the uterus if it is not too large.

PROLAPSE OF THE UTERUS

This condition results when the supporting structures of the uterus are weakened and the uterus collapses into the vagina. Prolapse of the uterus is sometimes associated with a cystocele, a rectocele, and an enterocele.

In cystocele, the bladder protrudes into the vaginal canal; in a rectocele, the rectum protrudes into the vaginal canal. In the total number of hysterectomies performed per year, prolapse of the uterus accounts for more than 35 percent and far exceeds myomas of the uterus.

Symptoms of Prolapse of the Uterus

A variety of symptoms result, such as pain with sexual intercourse, pelvic pressure, and, the most annoying of all symptoms, the inability to retain urine, or stress incontinence (urine flow following sneezing, coughing, or laughing). Repeated infections can result. Prolapse may become so severe that the uterus actually protrudes outside the vagina.

Pessaries (supporting instruments inserted into the vagina), formerly used, are no longer needed with the advent of superior surgical treatment.

The Controversy

When the gynecologist recommends surgery and the patient is asymptomatic, surgery need not be performed. The consensus of opinion is that surgery is indicated when symptoms become severe and intolerable.

When this repair is done on a young woman who desires to become pregnant again, the uterus needs to be left intact, recognizing that when the patient delivers, the repair will break down or it may be necessary to perform a Cesarean section.

Should the Ovaries Be Removed Along with the Uterus in This Situation?

This is one of the most controversial issues in gynecology and it arises whenever a noncancerous uterus is removed. It is a difficult decision to make and a second opinion is welcomed by the gynecologist. Once ovaries are removed, an artificial menopausal state is created: the woman may suffer unpleasant menopausal symptoms, such as hot flashes and some fatigue. Female hormones can correct these symptoms, but does the risk of breast cancer and heart disease justify their use? If the ovaries are left intact, there will be no menopausal symptoms, but there is the danger of cancer of the ovary in later years. Statistically, it is not known whether there is a greater risk of developing cancer of the intact ovary or a greater danger that a susceptibility to estrogen may lead to breast cancer and heart disease.

Here are some guidelines that may help make this decision:

A woman close to menopause—also a woman in her thirties with a strong family history of cancer—probably should also have her ovaries removed. A young woman with a negative family history probably should have her ovaries left intact.

Only after the patient has had a thorough discussion with her gynecologist and reached proper understanding of the situation should the decision be made.

CANCER OF THE CERVIX

This is largely a preventable disease. Cancer of the cervix (the structure described as the neck of the uterus opening into the vagina) is the second most invasive common form of cancer in America; there is an annual rate of twenty thousand cases, of whom seventy-five hundred will die.

Cancer of the cervix is unevenly distributed among certain groups. For example, Puerto Rican women have four times the incidence of this disease as mainland women. The black American is two and a half times more likely to have this cancer than the white woman. It is rare among Jewish women, and it has been theorized that circumcised males are less likely than other men to harbor and transmit a virus—if a virus causes cancer of the cervix. Having multiple sexual partners seems to lead to increased incidence of cancer of the cervix. Cancer of the uterine cervix is observed more often in women who have intercourse before the age of eighteen. It is nonexistent in nuns.

Carcinoma in Situ (Precancer)

This is 100 percent curable when the cancer cells occupy the outer layers of the cervix.

INCIDENCE

It is commonly found in menstruating females.

SYMPTOMS

There may be none. Minimal symptoms, such as longer menstrual periods, watery discharge, bleeding between periods, and a renewed bleeding after cessation of menses, may bring the patient to the doctor.

DIAGNOSIS

Often this cancer is found as a result of a routine pap smear and is considered a precancerous state. Untreated, it will progress to true invasive cancer in 75 percent of patients. Over fifty years ago George N. Papanicolaou observed that malignant cervical tumors shed cells which can be detected by the examination. It is still tragic that as recently as 1977 about seventy-five hundred American women died from cervical cancer, which could have been detected early and cured.

Once the pap smear identifies the abnormal cells, an iodine solution is spread over the cervix. Normal cervix tissue will be stained brown because it contains a sugar called glycogen. The region that contains the cancer cells remains unstained and the biopsy is taken in that area. Also, colposcopy will locate an abnormal surface area on the cervix. The colposcope is a special microscope that can magnify the cervix ten to twenty times. In Europe this has been a very popular method, in contrast to the United States, which is just starting to use this diagnostic system.

Cone Biopsy of the Cervix (Conization)

This procedure, in which part of the cervix is removed, is performed in the operating room under general anesthesia or spinal. A scalpel is used to "cone out" the inner part of the cervix, as one might remove the core of the apple. The biopsy actually removes the tumor. Subsequent follow-up is necessary, as this disease may recur. Some women prefer not to take the chance and elect to have a hysterectomy.

Treatment of Preinvasive Cancer or Cancer in Situ of the Cervix

As this condition may appear very often in women who are still in their late teens or early twenties and have not had any children, hysterectomy is not the preferred form of treatment. Another treatment besides hysterectomy is conization, just described. Sometimes the biopsy itself heals the patient. Electric cauterization of very localized lesions on the cervix is currently used, as is cryotherapy, which means destruction of the tumor by freezing.

Cryosurgery (Freezing)

A relatively recent procedure, widely used in the past ten years, cryosurgery is performed in the gynecologist's office. A probe is placed in the cervix and cooled to a freezing temperature by means of a cooling gas pumped through the instrument. The cells become frozen and are killed, and new normal cells now grow in the cervix. Careful follow-up is needed because the cancer cells can recur.

A young woman who wants to have children should not have a hysterectomy, but can choose between cryosurgery and cauterization. When precancer is found in someone who has already completed her family, gynecologists favor a hysterectomy, which will then relieve the woman of the constant dread of uterine cancer reappearing.

INVASIVE CANCER OF THE CERVIX

Diagnostic Examinations

After colposcopic examination and biopsy, staging of the lesion is essential to decide the type of treatment that will best benefit the patient. While in the hospital, the woman, under anesthesia, receives the same type of pelvic examination as in the gynecologist's office. It is much easier to do a more thorough examination with the patient under anesthesia. Special X rays are included: intravenous pyelogram to visualize the urinary tract, and a barium enema to see the colon. These X rays are performed to decide if the bladder and colon have been invaded by the cancer.

Staging of Cancer of the Cervix

Stage o cervical cancer, or carcinoma in situ (precancer), has already been discussed. Stage I cancer is confined strictly to the cervix and does not involve any part of the uterus or pelvic structure. Ninety percent of women will survive with treatment. External radiation with cobalt or radioactive radium or cesium implants is introduced through the vagina into the cervix and uterus and left in place for many hours, usually on two separate occasions about two weeks apart. The cure rate is the same whether surgery or radiation therapy is used. In young women radical hysterectomy with the biopsy of the ovaries for stage I disease is favored.

Stage II cancer extends beyond the cervix and up into the main body of the uterus, but has not spread to the wall of the pelvis. The vagina may be involved in its upper portion. Seventy percent of women survive stage II. The treatment is the same as for stage I, except no hysterectomy is performed.

Stage III cervical cancer has extended into the muscular wall surrounding the uterus and the vagina and the lower third of the vagina. Thirty-five percent of patients will survive this lesion after treatment. Therapy in this case is principally with external radiation, as the large bulky tumor mass makes an internal application of radioactive implants almost impossible.

Stage IV cervical cancer has invaded the bladder or rectum and extended beyond the limits of the pelvis. Survival with this extensive involvement is 14 percent and therapy is the same as in stage III, with the addition of chemotherapy.

Cancer of the Cervix Discovered During Pregnancy

If cancer is at Stage o, the pregnancy continues and therapy is undertaken afterward. If the cancer is more advanced, abortions are advised up to the twenty-fourth week, followed by treatment. When cancer is found after the twenty-fourth week, Cesarean section is performed, along with either a total hysterectomy or radiation.

Radiation Therapy

Radiation therapy is commonly used for the treatment of cervical cancer. A source of radiation (usually radium seeds) is placed in the vagina up against and within the cervix. This is left in place for a number of hours, the time being calculated to deliver a known amount of radiation to the cervix and nearby pelvic structures. Two radium applications are often used, and this is usually followed by a course of external radiation treatments. In these treatments a machine is used to deliver radiation to the pelvis in areas that could not be reached by the radium implanted in the vagina.

Radiation kills cells that are rapidly dividing, as in a malignancy. Current methods of radiation therapy are similar to surgery in their success rate in treating early stages of invasive cervical cancer. When the cancer has not spread beyond the cervix, the five-year "cure rate" is in the range of 95 percent, whether treatment is with surgery or radiation. With more advanced disease these five-year survival rates are lower. Often there is a ten-year survival rate.

Though the uterus and ovaries remain in place after radiation therapy, they are no longer able to function. Pregnancy is impossible; the ovaries stop releasing eggs and producing estrogen hormones. If menopause has not already occurred, it will occur at the time of treatment. A woman who has had radiation therapy for carcinoma of the cervix may continue to have a normal sexual life: there is no danger of her giving cancer to her sexual partner, as this is not a contagious disease. In fact, women who have had radiation therapy of this type are encouraged to resume sexual activity (once healing has occurred) in order to prevent the vagina from becoming narrowed because of scar-tissue formation. Despite these problems, there is low risk with radiation therapy, compared with its benefits for women with carcinoma of the cervix.

CANCER OF THE UTERINE BODY, OR ENDOMETRIAL CANCER

Warning Signs of Cancer of the Uterine Body, or Endometrial Cancer

1. Postmenopausal bleeding, regardless of amount.
2. Excessive bleeding or bleeding between menstruation in women approaching menopause.
3. Strong family history of cancer of the uterus, requiring careful and frequent gynecological examinations. Estrogens are to be avoided for menopausal symptoms.

Predisposition of This Cancer

Cancer of the glandular covering of the uterus, called the *endometrium,* is the most common cancer of the uterus. This is a cancer of an older age group than cervical cancer and the majority of women are past menopause. In contrast to cancer of the cervix, it is common in Jewish women and in women who have no children. Certain women—those who are obese and have high levels of estrogens—are more likely to develop cancer of the uterus. This cancer is also found more often in women who have a family history of uterine cancer, and a long history of irregular bleeding, skipping periods, and who have had several D & Cs.

Endometrial Hyperplasia

This condition, resulting from excessive estrogen stimulation, causes glandular overgrowth of the endometrium, commonly showing up in women who are about to go through menopause. Some gynecologists report this condition as the forerunner of cancer of the uterus. It is diagnosed with a D & C. Depending on the pathology found, either a hysterectomy or hormonal treatment (progesterone) is advised.

The Diagnosis of Uterine Cancer or Endometrial Cancer

Every year twenty-eight thousand American women are found to have endometrial cancer, of whom three to four thousand will die. We want to emphasize again that early discovery makes it possible to cure this malignancy. The only effective and correct way to diagnose this illness is by a D & C (dilatation and curettage). Microscopic examination of the specimen will make this diagnosis firm. The pelvic examination might reveal a very large, boggy uterus. The worst finding is positive cancer cells in the vagina, as the patient with this condition will rarely survive five years.

The survival rate for early-diagnosed cases of uterine cancer is very good, usually 90 percent or more, but, if the wall of the uterus is invaded by tumor, the survival rate drops to 70 percent, and if the tumor extends down to the cervix, only 50 percent will be cured.

Treatment of Cancer of the Uterus

If the patient is elderly, then nonsurgical treatment with radiation therapy alone may be indicated. Younger patients in which the cancer has not spread have radiation first, followed by a radical abdominal hysterectomy with removal of the ovaries and the tubes. In the past surgeons also removed all the lymph nodes, but there is no evidence that this increases the overall survival rate.

Radiation given before surgery is administered by means of small radioactive seeds called *Heyman capsules*. These are introduced through the vagina and left in place for three days.

Numerous studies have demonstrated that internal radiation is the best method. In advanced cancer of the uterus with spread of the tumor cells to the lungs and other organs, when the patient is inoperable, hormonal treatment is used.

The hormone progesterone, which is normally secreted in small quantities by the ovaries during the menstrual cycle, prepares the uterine lining for implantation of the fertilized egg. Progesterone causes shrinking of the tumor deposits and may actually melt away the deposits in the lung. Patients who have been suffering and are critically ill report a decrease in pain and a sense of well-being. The complication of progesterone treatment is primarily related to the heart. If the patient has heart disease, it may worsen the cardiac condition by causing the patient to retain water, placing an even greater load on the heart.

CANCER OF THE OVARY

These egg-shaped organs produce female hormones—estrogens and progesterones—and are the most deceptive of all organs. They are so well sheltered within the pelvic cavity that many times discovery of cancer is a belated event. The ovary, like the rest of the female system, has been the object of myths and false speculations. It was thought in medieval medicine that the ovaries were filled with semen, and that it was there that semen was formed and spread down into the tubes—labeled spermatic vessels—to the horns of the uterus. It took Gabriel Fallopius to describe and put into clear perspective the ovary and its tubes; his famous observation was published in Venice in 1561, a year before his death.

One of the most bizarre reasons for operating on the ovary occurred in the 1800s. It was then believed that a condition called ovariomania, known today as nymphomania, could only be cured by the removal of the ovary. Furthermore, masturbation was also considered to be treatable with the removal of the ovary along with mixtures of bromides, chlorides, and hydrochloride of cocaine.

Cancer of the ovary is a discouraging illness for the patient and the gynecologist. The only way to reduce the incidence of this disease is by routine removal of the ovaries on any woman undergoing a hysterectomy. This is acceptable for women forty-five years of age or older, but not a universal practice in women below that age. The pap smear is ineffective in locating disease of the ovaries, but a thorough pelvic examination may pick up abnormalities. This is considered the third most common female malignancy, and results in the largest number of deaths.

Despite the advances in surgery and radiation, only 30 percent of women manage to survive. There are surveys in Connecticut which disclose a 15 percent increase in cancer of the ovary. The incidence of this cancer increases with age: ten cases per thousand are reported yearly for women thirty-five to thirty-eight years of age; between the ages of sixty-five to sixty-nine, fifty women per one thousand are afflicted.

The Symptoms of Cancer of the Ovary

Symptoms may consist primarily of pressure symptoms, which may be minimal, but as the cancer involves the digestive system, complaints such as bloating, cramps, and nausea may occur. A large mass can fill the entire pelvis, simulating a pregnant uterus. As the tumor cells implant into the covering of the digestive organs, fluid may accumulate, causing gigantic swelling or ascites.

Diagnosis of Cancer of the Ovary

The diagnosis of ovarian cancer can only be established with certainty by opening the abdomen and removing tissue for diagnosis. Today, ultrasonography is being used to diagnose ovarian tumors and cysts. It is simple, with no risks, and can be repeated numerous times. Accurate interpretation by a radiologist specially trained for this procedure is essential or misdiagnosis can occur. It is helpful but not conclusive and the diagnosis can only be clearly made by opening the abdomen.

Treatment of Cancer of the Ovary

The treatment, except in far-advanced cases, is surgery with the removal of the uterus, the ovaries, and the fallopian tubes. If the tumor is too large, radiation treatment is given first and then an operation is performed.

Medical treatment, chemotherapy, is playing an important role in ovarian cancers. Oncologists report some miraculous results, and, in some cases, cure. In the future the treatment of cancer of the ovary will probably be primarily chemotherapy, as surgery and radiotherapy will be little used. At the present time there is a great deal of research on drugs that will effectively alter the course and cure of cancer of the ovaries.

Cysts of the Ovary

During a routine gynecological examination the physician might feel one or both of the ovaries to be enlarged and suggest an exploratory operation and possible hysterectomy with removal of the ovaries. The patient may want a second opinion in this case. Enlargement of the ovaries can occur during a menstrual cycle and then may regress in size as menstruation begins. The mass the physician feels may indeed be a tumor or a cyst.

Part of the examination should include ultrasonography. The "echo" of the abdomen needs to be performed by an expert trained in ultrasonography. If the echo finds no cyst and the physician still feels one, a second opinion may be helpful: either the echo reading is incorrect or there really is no cyst. This dilemma occurs much too frequently in practice to ignore.

Another echo may need to be done at a different institution and with a different gynecologist. It may be that the cyst comes and goes according to the menstrual cycle.

When the clinician and the echo agree, then surgery may be indicated. If more than one physician feels the cyst and the echo does not demonstrate the cyst, surgery should also be considered. Nothing is as accurate as the experience of a good gynecologist who has a long track record of proper diagnoses. After all, ultrasonography is still a new test and many more years of experience are necessary before its validity can be completely justified.

Removal of a Normal Uterus

Every organ that is removed in a hospital is sent to the pathologist for examination. Very often a uterus examined by the pathologist is considered to be normal. Normal uteruses are often removed for prolapse, which we have discussed, or when both ovaries are diseased and the uterus is removed at the same time.

Normal uteruses are also removed to achieve sterilization and there are several circumstances when this is indicated. Menstrual periods are a traumatic event for mentally retarded patients, and hysterectomy will often be performed in these circumstances. Family histories that are very strong in cancers of the uterus may also be an indication.

Adenomyosis

This is another reason for performing a hysterectomy. This disease affects women in their thirties and forties. It is a benign disease of the uterus.

PATHOLOGY

The cavity of the uterus is lined with specialized tissue, the endometrium, which sheds every month at the time of a menstrual period if the woman is not pregnant. Adenomyosis means the endometrium has now penetrated into the actual muscular wall of the uterus, sending fingerlike projections into the wall. It is found most frequently in women who have had several pregnancies and is associated with fibroids.

THE SYMPTOMS OF ADENOMYOSIS

The outstanding symptoms may be painful intercourse and very painful menstrual periods that continue throughout the month. Menopause relieves the patient with this illness, but the only definitive treatment is hysterectomy.

The physical examination will disclose a uterus that is twice the normal size. Menstrual periods become so painful that patients resort to painkillers, at first prescribed by their physicians. One of the complications of this illness is drug addiction. It is hard to know how many women are hooked on pain medications such as codeine. At one time, especially in Europe, medications combined with aspirin, phenacetin, and phenobarbital could be purchased over the counter. In clinical practice patients were seen, and are still seen today, who are dependent on these medications. Only after a very thorough history is taken by the medical doctor will this diagnosis be made.

Hysterectomy is indicated when the condition becomes intolerable and there is danger of drug addiction.

Endometriosis

This is the most painful disease of the female organs. The cause is unknown, but some doctors feel it is the result of menstrual blood flowing back into the pelvic cavity. The greatest incidence of the disease is seen in women under thirty, it is more common in white women than in black women, and is relieved by pregnancy.

PATHOLOGY OF ENDOMETRIOSIS

In this condition the endometrium wanders outside of the uterus. This is not a cancerous condition, although in some

Summation of Questions and Results of Hysterectomy
500 Patients *

QUESTION	%
Are you pleased you had a hysterectomy?	
Yes	90.9
No	2.9
Blank	5.1
Not sure	1.1
Would you encourage a friend to proceed with or postpone hysterectomy?	
Proceed	84.7
Postpone	4.4
Depends on circumstances	3.6
Blank or neither	7.3
When fully recovered, did you feel better or worse than before?	
Better	77.8
Worse	4.0
Both of the above	12.8
Same	4.7
Blank	0.7
In what way did you feel better?	
Less inconvenience	69.7
More energy	53.7
Better sex life	38.0
No more (or less) pain	14.6
Better emotionally	7.7
Better generally	7.3
No dyspareunia	4.0
No more fear of pregnancy	1.5
No fear of cancer	0.4
Less discharge	0.4
Saved my life	0.4
Bowels better	0.4
No fear of oral contraceptives	0.4
In what way did you feel worse?	
Weight gain	8.8
Worse sex life	6.2
Depression	5.1
Weight loss	2.6

Question	%
Tired, less energy	1.1
Bladder problems	0.4
Menopause symptoms	0.4
Loss of muscle control	0.4
Still have pain	0.4
Was your hysterectomy elective?	
Yes	69.7
No	29.6
Not sure	0.7
Was your hysterectomy (if elective) unnecessary?	
No	92.8
Yes	2.8
Not sure	3.3
Blank	1.1
Were you aware of the risks inherent in hysterectomy?	
Yes	90.5
No	7.7
Not sure	1.1
Some	0.4
No risk	0.4
Do you feel that you needed a second opinion to help you decide whether or not you wished to have surgery? Did you get one?	
Needed	32.5
Sought	39.1
Blank	0.4
No to both questions	56.6

*Reprinted with permission from Bruce C. Richards, M.D., and the C.V. Mosby Co., from: *Hysterectomy: From Women to Women,* Am J Obstet Gynecol 131:4, 1978

ways it behaves like one because it spreads and infiltrates other organs. The tissue of the endometrium can penetrate into the appendix, the colon, and even the bladder.

THE SYMPTOMS OF ENDOMETRIOSIS

The disease may manifest itself with severe pain during menstruation and sexual intercourse. Careful history will reveal that some patients have painful bowel movements during menstrual periods or recurrent severe pain in the abdomen which can simulate appendicitis, gallbladder disease, or colitis. It may also penetrate the ovaries and destroy them. This disease continues and progresses as long as the ovaries are functioning. Sometimes these patients may present with recurrent symptoms that are interpreted as emotional and are referred to a psychiatrist.

The diagnosis should be preceded by careful history and sometimes a D & C will confirm it.

The Treatment of Endometriosis

The only way to be certain of curing this illness is to remove the uterus and ovaries. When the patient wishes to have children, conservative surgery removing the endometrial implants is used.

Medical treatment is sometimes tried with oral contraceptive pills with moderate success.

The diagnosis is generally made with the aid of a laparoscope, a simple instrument which is much like a telescope and is designed to look into the pelvis. Endometriosis is not a precancerous condition. Cysts of the ovary, called chocolate cysts, may occur from endometriosis. They are so called because they contain a thick dark-brown fluid resembling liquid chocolate; the color is the result of bleeding into the cyst. When these cysts rupture, they can cause a severe emergency with acute abdominal pain, called peritonitis.

Second opinions are needed before elective surgical hysterectomies are performed. It is hoped that unnecessary surgery would be eliminated and millions of dollars saved. Here is a quote from the American College of Obstetrics and Gynecology:

> The clinical findings in many of the conditions for which surgery
> is advisable are specific. Unfortunately, the clinical findings of other
> conditions may not be nearly so conclusive. The evaluation by sev-

eral physicians of patients with conditions may result in different recommendations for treatment.

The evaluation by the physician should include the "total" patient. Such an evaluation is especially important for the problems which are not associated with clear-cut pathologic findings but which may seriously affect the quality of life for the patient. For such problems the recommendations of the physician who has known the individual for many years are much more likely to be correct than the recommendations of a similarly qualified physician who has seen the patient only once or twice.

A consultation with one or more physicians is often desirable. The attending physician may request such consultations because of preexisting conditions which are outside his or her area of expertise or because of developing complications. Consultations may also be sought by thoroughly competent physicians regarding the care of patients who have unusually serious conditions or complications.

The patient may request the opinions of one or more additional physicians. Such requests should be encouraged and honored.

CESAREAN SECTION

It was during an evening TV news broadcast, in which the broadcaster intimated that incidence of Cesarean section was rapidly increasing and that doctors use Cesarean section to shorten delivery time and increase their fees, that the authors were prompted to include a discussion of Cesarean section in this book. Statistically the number of Cesarean sections has remained rather constant in the past ten years, reported as 35 percent. The pregnant woman now armed with consumer and government reports questions the procedure and the scientific justification.

By Cesarean section we are referring to an operation for the removal of a fetus from the uterus by an abdominal incision. It is a myth that Julius Caesar was born in this way. Pompilius, ruler of Rome from 715 to 673 B.C., decreed if any woman died while she was pregnant, the child would immediately be cut out of her abdomen. This was part of the Lex Regia, which, under the emperors, became the Lex Caesare, and the operation was known as the Cesarean operation or section.

Removal of a dead fetus was done either manually or by inserting hooks. Decapitation was necessary in some cases and this was affected by means of a hook with a sharpened curve. In 1608 the Senate in Venice proclaimed that any practitioner who failed to perform this operation on a dead pregnant woman laid himself open to very heavy penalties. The first legendary Cesarean section was Apollo's removal of the body of Asclepius from the womb of the dead Coronis. Bacchus was supposed to have been brought into the world in the same manner. The earliest suggestion that the operation might have been performed with success on a living woman is not Roman but Jewish and occurs in that part of the Talmud called the Mishna. The first recorded incidence of a Cesarean being performed on a living woman occurred about 1500 when a Swiss pig gelder operated on his own wife.

Indications for Cesarean Section

The most common reasons for doing a primary Cesarean section is when the fetus is in a grossly abnormal position and vaginal delivery would not be possible. Forty percent of all first Cesarean sections were done because the fetus would not fit through the pelvis. Some institutions report an increase in indications from primary Cesarean sections as accurate new ways are developed for measuring fetal distress through fetal heart-rate monitoring.

If during the course of a delivery the fetal heart is distressed, Cesarean section needs to be performed to save the baby. Other indications of breech presentation or the sitting position have increased significantly in the past ten years. Primary Cesarean section for breech presentation has increased from 12 percent to 21 percent. If the increase of Cesarean sections is reported by some institutions, it is because of the increase of breech presentation and of the greater ability to identify fetal distress.

Other situations necessitating Cesarean sections are bleeding in the last three months of pregnancy, and a uterus that loses its contractile force even after it is induced with medication called Pitocin. Also included are prolapse of the umbilical cord through the uterus, previous Cesarean sections, and apparent catastrophic illnesses of the fetus, such as erythroblastosis, which requires immediate exchange transfusions.

Cesarean sections are performed, for the most part, to help the baby survive and, in some instances, to save the mother. Contrary to public editorials, the reasons why Cesarean sections are increasing is because of the identification of the abnormalities described. It seems evident that more infants are surviving the prenatal period and that the quality of their life has been significantly improved. Long-term disabilities resulting from severe forms of brain damage are decreased. Undoubtedly, Cesarean section is one of the contributing factors.

Vaginal delivery remains the safest method of delivery for the mother and child, and only after increased risk has been carefully documented should a Cesarean section be performed. We fully agree a Cesarean section should not be performed for the convenience of the gynecologist to hurry the delivery along, but only for the safety of the mother and the fetus.

5: Kidney Stones

"OH LORD, TAKE ME NOT THROUGH THE KIDNEY." So lamented Sir Jonathan Hutchinson of Yorkshire, surgeon to the London Hospital in 1875. Sir Jonathan was referring to one of the most painful conditions in medicine—the kidney stone.

The oldest renal stone was recovered from an Egyptian mummy dated seven thousand years old. According to Marco Polo, the Khan of Mongolia, named Kublai, suffered from gout and kidney stones in the year 1267. Some medical historians feel Alexander the Great made a serious military blunder during the Persian War because he suffered from an attack of gout and kidney stones. John Milton's *Paradise Lost* was allegedly written at the time when he was suffering from stone disease.

Folklore has developed around such stones since antiquity. For example, kidney stones worn around the neck were used to ward off hysteria, prevent melancholy, and treat poisons from snakebite.

It has been estimated that in the United States kidney-stone disease accounts for 200,000 hospitalized patients per year.

This figure does not include the numerous office and emergency room visits by patients suffering from kidney-stone attacks (renal colic). Epidemics have occurred in various countries, most notably in England in the late eighteenth century, when one in every thirty-eight patients hospitalized had renal-stone disease. Similar episodes appear today to involve male children in Southeast Asia and India.

The Cause of Kidney Stones

There is still much speculation about the cause as well as the mechanism of stone formation. Among the factors mentioned by kidney specialists are diet, type of water drunk, climate, and environment. As an example, in 1931 a scientist by the name of Jolly made the observation that stones are most common in areas where the inhabitants subsist on diets composed mostly of cereal grains. Epidemiological evidence and historical observation have found the incidence of stone disease higher among relatives of stone formers.

The Physiology of Stone Formation

The most common varieties of kidney stones are 1) calcium stones, 2) mixed calcium stones with magnesium, ammonia, and phosphate, 3) uric acid stones, and 4) cystine stones. Other types which are very rare need not be mentioned.

CALCIUM STONES AND MIXED STONES

The most common stone formation in the United States contains calcium and oxalate and/or phosphate, making up 75 percent of the stone population of this country. These stones are most common, by far, in men in the third to fifth decades of life. Another medical mystery that confounds doctors is why calcium stones are more common in "stone belts," as, for example, in the southeast portion of the United States. Calcium stone formation may occur as a complication of a variety of illnesses. An overactive parathyroid gland, which governs calcium metabolism, may cause stone formation.

People who develop calcium stones may have parents and grandparents who were "stone people." Patients who just do not drink enough fluid and pass a small volume of urine, if they have a predisposition for calcium stone formation, may form stones. Food faddists ingesting excessive amounts of vitamins, especially vitamins A and D, have an increased incidence of recurrent kidney stones and kidney disease. High dosages of vitamin C (more than 4 grams per day) can also lead to stones.

URIC ACID STONE DISEASE

Uric acid is the product of the normal metabolism of the body. After uric acid is formed, it is excreted by the kidney into the urine. When there is too much uric acid manufactured, and/or too much excreted by the kidney, it accumulates in the urine and causes stones. In some people excess uric acid becomes deposited in joints, causing the familiar disease called gout. Stones found in Egyptian mummies were of the uric acid type. Ten percent of stones found in the United States are composed of uric acid. Uric acid stones tend to form when the urine is concentrated, which means that the patient has not been drinking enough water and there is too much acid in the urine.

CYSTINE STONES

These account for 1 or 2 percent of kidney stones detected in patients in the United States. Cystine is produced by the body from metabolism of proteins and should be normally retained in the body. When the kidneys fail to retain cystine, it appears in the urine and can form stones, especially if the urine is too acid and too concentrated.

Kidney stones represent an aberration in the normal metabolism of the body. Calcium is the basic element needed for our bony structures. Too much of this substance causes kidney stones and other complications. It is an amazing trick of nature how things are in constant balance, or homeostasis. A slight molecular change in the composition of the normal elements in our bodies can have devastating effects, such as stone formation.

Anatomy of the Urinary Tract

Waste products are eliminated from the body through the bowel and through the urinary tract. A right and left kidney take the waste products from the blood and pass them through tubes called the ureters. The adult ureter, measuring approximately 30 cm long and following a rather gentle S curve, empties into the urinary bladder. The bladder is a hollow muscular organ which serves as a reservoir for urine. It has a capacity of approximately 400 to 500 cm of urine. The adult bladder lies behind the front arch of the pelvis and empties from the body through the urethra. In the male the urethra lies in the shaft of the penis and is 8 to 15 cm long. In the female it is approximately 3 cm long and is slightly curved and lies behind the pelvis just in the front portion of the vagina.

Symptoms of Kidney Stones

Once having had a kidney-stone attack, or witnessing the poor soul afflicted with this whipping pain, a person will never mistake it for anything else. The onset of the pain may be insidious, with a little discomfort in the abdomen, lasting but a few seconds and then it may return with a startling, excruciating knifelike pain that takes one's very breath away. The patient bends over or may roll on the floor, clutching his abdomen, twisting his body in agonizing fear, crying out, as he swiftly becomes drenched in sweat. The pain may subside spontaneously, but reappear a few minutes later. The patient assumes bizarre, twisted postures, as he can't lie still. The pain may proceed down from the abdomen, reaching toward the genitals. In the emergency room the patient presents with an unmistakable picture and requires morphine, sometimes in repeated dosages, to get relief. So characteristic is the pain that drug addicts capitalize on the symptoms with the emergency room staff, begging for morphine to relieve their fictitious pain.

The pain may subside spontaneously or continue for hours as the stone travels from the kidney through the narrow passage of the ureter. With good fortune the stone may travel down out of the urinary tract, and as the patient urinates, he hears that precious jingling sound of the stone striking the bottom of the toilet bowl—the sound that the attack is over until the next time.

No wonder Sir Sidney, a clergyman of the 1820s, once described a kidney stone pain "as if somebody is walking on my eyeballs," or, in the same breath, he announced, "put my hand in a vise and turn it thrice and then make three more turns and you will know the pain of a kidney stone."

During his attacks Benjamin Franklin stood on his head to urinate to avoid having his stone fall into the urethral opening. In this position he discovered he could release the stone. He invented his own urinary catheter, which he shared with his brother, to release the stone.

Amongst other sufferers of the stone disease was the French essayist, Montaigne, who wrote: "I feel everywhere, men tormented with the same disease: and am honored by the fellowship, for as much as men of the best quality are most frequently afflicted with it; 'tis a noble and dignified disease. Were it not a good office to a man to put him in mind of his end? My kidneys claw me to purpose."

Cicero also had kidney stones and reported that he eliminated stones at night while dreaming of a beautiful woman.

When stones are "of the silent variety," they do not present with symptoms of pain but are found incidentally during a routine X-ray examination.

The Diagnosis of Kidney Stones

By getting a careful history, or actually observing a kidney-stone attack (called renal colic), the physician can easily make the diagnosis. It is crucial to attempt to recover the stone that has passed in the urine in order to identify its chemical composition.

X-ray examinations are included in the diagnostic workup, called *intravenous pyelogram*. Calcium stones are easily visualized by plain X-ray films, while pure uric acid stones are not seen by ordinary X-ray examination. X rays are essential, not only for the identification of the stone, but to determine if the stone has caused any obstruction of the urine flow. If obstruction occurs, some of the 400 to 1500 cm of urine formed each day will be prevented from being eliminated and an actual backing-up of the urine into one of the kidneys may occur, causing injury to the organ.

THE INTRAVENOUS PYELOGRAM

The intravenous pyelogram, also referred to as IVP, is a method of X-ray visualization of the structures within the kidney, the ureters, and the bladder. An iodine-containing dye is injected into a vein and is carried by the blood to the kidneys. Five minutes after the injection of the dye, X rays are taken, and then another set is taken at ten minutes, and another at about fifteen minutes. Prior to this examination the intestine must be cleared with strong laxatives so the kidney X ray can be taken without being obscured by gas and fluid in the bowel.

The danger of the intravenous pyelography is reaction to the dye. Patients who are known to be allergic to iodine products, fish, or the dye itself should notify their physician of their allergic history and question the advisability of an IVP. Prior to

doing the intravenous pyelogram, the radiologist should in-
quire as to whether the patient has any allergy to fish or iodine.

CYSTOSCOPIC EXAMINATION

An instrument called a *cystoscope* is passed into the bladder
through the urethra. Through the cystoscope, stones and
foreign bodies can be removed, as well as biopsies taken. This is
not a particularly painful procedure, but it does cause considerable anxiety, especially among male patients. There is a minimal risk of damage, and, occasionally, infections may occur.

The physician looks through the cystoscope to examine the
interior of the urethra and bladder. This is commonly performed in the urologist's office, either under local or general
anesthesia. The area around the genitals is cleaned with an antiseptic solution. The cystoscope is lubricated and then slowly
passed through the urethra and into the bladder. A sterile fluid
may be introduced into the bladder through the cystoscope.
This fluid serves to stretch out the walls of the bladder so that
the physician can get a clearer view.

This examination should be reserved for episodes of recurrent stones, if obstruction is suspected, and for unexplained
blood in the urine. Fortunately, most patients have one kidney-
stone attack in a lifetime and need not be cystoscoped.

LABORATORY TESTS

Blood chemistries must be performed to determine the level
of calcium and uric acid in the blood. An adequate history must
also be taken on the dietary consumption and the amount of
fluid intake and medications which the patient may be taking.
A thorough family history is also necessary to identify "stone
families." A urine culture must be performed in order to identify patients in whom infection may be contributing to stone
formation. In addition, a twenty-four-hour urine collection for

measurement of calcium and uric acid must be done, as well as screening for cystine.

Sometimes the patient may present with a history suggestive of a kidney stone, but it cannot be demonstrated either by X-ray findings or urine examination. This circumstance may occur if the patient has passed the stone. The doctor who specializes in the diagnosis and treatment of kidney stones works closely with the medical doctor to solve the mystery of the missing stone and its composition. Sometimes the stone is never identified. It is inadequate to make a diagnosis of kidney stone without attempting to find its composition and cause. The doctor will instruct the patient to filter his urine through a urinary strainer. The simplest method is to take a paper towel and pass urine through it.

Medical Treatment of Stones

The patient should seek a second opinion if the physician does not make a heroic attempt to identify the cause and identity of the stone. The treatment of kidney stones is a combined effort of the medical man and the surgeon. The medical man is needed because kidney stones, after all, are frequently the result of a metabolic disorder with surgical consequences. The type of stone discovered will determine what is the best treatment. For example, if a uric acid stone is identified and the patient has a markedly elevated uric acid in his blood and urine, the medication allopurinol (Zyloprim) can be used to reduce formation of uric acid and can occasionally actually dissolve kidney stones by absorption of calcium through the intestines.

Maintenance of a diluted urine is the mainstay of treatment of all urinary stones. To maintain a continuous flow of dilute urine, an adult must urinate approximately 3 to 4 quarts of urine in twenty-four hours. In many cases this method alone, if conscientiously followed, keeps stones from forming or at least decreases the rate at which they form and pass. A drug, called a thiazide diuretic, is currently used for calcium-stone formers who have a high calcium in their urine. These measures must be used along with the surgical procedure. In spite of all these excellent measures, stones may continue to form, to the frustration of the patient and doctor.

The Surgical Treatment of Kidney Stones

The removal of stones from the bladder is one of the oldest forms of surgery recorded in the history of medicine. Lithotomy, or cutting for stones, was used during the dynasties of Egypt and reached its height in the seventeenth and eighteenth centuries in England and France when silver and woven silk catheters were devised.

The first and foremost lithotomist was a nonmedical man by the name of Baulot, who was a medical assistant. He decided to go his own way, traveling throughout Europe. His reputation was so great that he was summoned to the royal courts of Europe with his fur-lined bag, displaying the different sizes of catheters, corresponding to the displayed urethral opening that he scrupulously inspected. The "lithotomy room" was devised as a torture chamber when not in use to clear the stone. Still, today, the catheter remains a noble, indispensable instrument to remove a stone from the urinary tract.

Premature attempts in trying to dislodge a stone are condemned by most surgeons. Early and repeated surgical manipulations increase risks and complications, such as infections, perforations, future scarring, and narrowing of the ureter.

After waiting forty-eight to seventy-two hours, if a stone has not passed spontaneously, as determined by the patient's continued pain and/or repeated X-ray films (the stone has moved down the long ureter tract but is still caught), the surgeon then should perform cystoscopy and, if possible, a "basket extraction." A *basket extraction* means that the end of the catheter is like a small basket that opens around the stone and closes as it is pulled out. If the intravenous pyelogram does not visualize the kidney, it could imply the stone has caused a complete obstruction of urine flow and the kidney will soon swell and may become injured unless the obstruction is promptly relieved.

Not all stones need to be removed. For example, stones that are less than 5 to 6 mm in diameter and that show movement between the first and repeated X-ray films (the first X-ray films being taken at the time of the attack and repeat films taken twenty-four and forty-eight hours later) are best left alone. About 90 percent may pass spontaneously, if not in the first two days of hospitalization, then within two to three weeks.

If pain continues or fever accompanies the acute obstruction, or both, a catheter should be passed into the ureter and left in place for a period of forty-eight hours. This dilates the ureter and may allow the stone to pass within a few days. If the pain is not too severe, the surgeon may choose to have the patient stay at home, giving him ample painkilling medications and instructions to increase his urinary output and filter his urine to find the stone, and treat with antibiotics for infections.

Stones larger than 5 to 6 mm in diameter are not likely to pass spontaneously, and, again, with repeated X rays, if they show no signs of progress and remain stuck in the middle or upper part of the ureter, surgical intervention is mandatory. If the stones of 5 to 6 mm are already in the end of the ureter, these can be removed by simple basket extraction in as many as 90 percent of cases. Stones remaining in the bladder are removed mechanically.

Silent kidney stones, which are not causing any urinary obstruction, are best left alone.

The important reminder is to keep the urine as dilute as possible, which is accomplished by increasing the fluid intake, especially at night. Dietary changes are sometimes helpful. For example, patients who have too much calcium in their urine can eliminate milk and milk products. In patients with normal calcium, this maneuver seems to be of little help. Recently the use of a thiazide diuretic reducing urine calcium excretion has received some support.

As to the future, we can look for the removal of stones by sonar, which is currently being tested, and perhaps more dietary manipulations and future medications will prevent the treacherous stone from forming.

6: Prostatic Surgery

THE PROSTATE GLAND, a necessary vital organ during the reproductive period of a man's life, may become an albatross in later
years. This gland, which is snugly located behind the pubis,
weighs about 30 grams, surrounds a short length of the
urethra, and contains the ejaculatory glands. Behind it is the
rectum, in front of it is the bony pubis. It is the fluid from
the prostate which gives lubrication and mobility to the sperm.

When the prostate gland enlarges, it presses on the outlet of
the urinary bladder and interferes with urination. The condition, called *benign hypertrophy of the prostate,* is a nonmalignant
overgrowth.

Causes for Benign Prostatic Enlargement

The causes of this condition are unknown. At one time doctors thought this illness due to either excessive sexual activity
or lack of it. Neither of these is even a casual factor. The
Bedouins (Arab nomads) rarely develop prostatic enlargement

because their prostates atrophy from horseback and camel riding.

Symptoms of Benign Prostatic Enlargement

There may be no initial complaints or the male may complain of embarrassing symptoms, such as taking a long time to urinate, dribbling, incontinence, and having to awaken several times during the night to empty his bladder. Sometimes the obstruction may be to such an extent that urination ceases completely. The urinary bladder then distends and actually can be felt as a swelling in the lower abdomen, causing the patient much grief and discomfort if the obstruction is not relieved. A continual, peristent, agonizing pain can follow and the bladder can, on rare occasions, actually rupture.

Beyond the age of sixty-five most men will have some degree of urinary obstruction. Impotence is not a symptom of prostatic enlargement.

Diagnosis of Prostatic Gland Benign Enlargement

Rectal examination will help diagnose an enlarged prostate gland. Sometimes the prostate may be enlarged and not within reach of the finger. Then cystoscopic examination is necessary to confirm the diagnosis.

Indications for Surgery

If retention of urine occurs acutely, a polyethylene catheter is inserted through the penis to empty the bladder. If the symptoms of increasing frequent urination, hesitation, post-dribbling, and retention persist, surgery is indicated.

A urologist, after a careful examination of a prostate, will also measure the amount of urine that is retained in the bladder after voiding. If a large volume of urine remains in the bladder, then this, too, is an indication for doing a prostate operation.

The History of Prostatic Surgery

This is another fascinating vignette worthy of recounting. In 1890 Hugh Hampton Young, the founder of modern urology, while still a surgical resident, treated a black man who arrived at the hospital in kidney failure because of severe prostatic enlargement. A catheter could not be passed through the penis into the bladder to drain it. Dr. Young made an incision into the lower abdomen to allow urine to drain, and in a few days the patient improved. He then stuck his finger into the bladder through the abdominal wall and shelled out the enormous prostate, signaling the first successful prostate operation. Dr. Young also became famous for treating James Brady, better known as Diamond Jim, for his prostate. Diamond Jim consulted Dr. Young because his general medical condition was so serious—he had diabetes, heart disease, and high blood pressure—that he could not have his prostate removed through the abdomen. Dr. Young had just devised an instrument so that the operation could be performed through the penis with a simple device called the prostatic punch. This operation, the first of its kind, is called *transurethral resection.* Added to his credits, Dr. Hugh Young also treated President Woodrow Wilson when the president was in urinary retention, after he had had a stroke.

Still, today, the prostate gland is removed surgically by three methods: one is called the *suprapubic prostatectomy* (Young's first operation); the second is called the *retropubic prostatectomy.* Both operations still involve the removal of the prostate through the lower abdomen. The retropubic approach is favored by most surgeons today as there is less bleeding. The third operation, transurethral resection (Diamond Jim's operation), consists of removing part of the gland blocking the urethra. The abdomen need not be opened, as the operation is performed through the penis.

In these operations the entire prostate gland is not removed but only partially removed. It has been described by some surgeons as "the removal of an egg, leaving the shell in place."

A relatively young patient with a very large prostate is generally operated on through the abdominal approach, but this entails a higher risk of complications and death.

The Medical Opinion

Operations should only be performed if the patient's symptoms become intolerable: hesitancy of urination, frequency of urination, inability to empty the bladder, and interference with normal sleep. The surgeon must be certain that the symptoms are coming from a benign hypertrophy of the prostate and not from an infection of the prostate, called *prostatitis*. Prostatitis can resemble an enlarged prostate. A prostate that is only slightly enlarged can become grossly enlarged if it becomes infected. Unnecessary surgery can be prevented if the diagnosis of prostatitis is ruled out by proper digital examination.

Patients who are confined to bed for even brief periods of time may develop prostate trouble, with the prostate becoming boggy and swollen, or infected. The insertion of a urinary catheter, leaving it in place for a short period of time, may allow the prostate to shrink back to the size it was before the infection.

The patient should ask the surgeon if his prostate is only infected and not enlarged, and whether a trial of antimicrobal therapy should be used before surgery is indicated. In most instances the surgeon will be able to tell the difference between the two conditions.

Prostatic massage and examination of the fluid which is expressed from the penis is helpful in diagnosing prostatitis. Sometimes, because of lack of sexual intercourse, acute congestion of the prostate may result, simulating prostatic benign hypertrophy of the prostate. The prostate then becomes swollen and moderately tender. Massage of the prostate will produce copious secretions with prompt cessation of symptoms.

Although the mortality of prostatic surgery is low, the complications may be many. These complications may consist of a generalized severe infection, hemorrhage, pulmonary embolism (clot to the lung), and a myocardial infarction. Patients with limited life expectancy can be relieved with no surgery by placing a permanent indwelling catheter. For example, elderly patients from nursing homes with diffuse cancer should not be subjected to surgery and should demand an alternative: permanent catheter placement.

Cancer of the Prostate

Once, during medical teaching rounds, an intern presented a patient to the professor of medicine. The patient complained of pain in his lower leg. This bright young doctor gave a detailed history of how this seventy-nine-year-old elderly gentleman, always in good health, suddenly developed severe pain in his leg and went to see his family doctor and an orthopedic surgeon and finally came to the university diagnostic clinic for an appraisal of his problems. A detailed description of the physical examination was given by the intern for the professor. At the end of the description, the professor asked the student, "And what did the rectal examination show?"

Blushing and embarrassed, the medical student stammered that he did not perform a rectal examination as the elderly gentleman was in such despair and pain that he thought this was not an essential part of the examination.

The professor, in an angry tone, replied, "Young man, if you don't put your finger in, you will have your foot in it later on."

The professor then proceeded to do a rectal examination, and, with a grim face, found a classical cancer of the prostate.

This anecdote describes accurately the dilemma of prostatic cancer, which accounts for seventeen thousand deaths per year and is the second leading cause of cancer deaths among elderly American men. What is even more alarming is that 30 percent, or twelve thousand of the new cases, are potentially curable when and if they are discovered.

SYMPTOMS

The cancer is found in many instances after it has spread (metastasized) to different parts of the body, especially to bone. The only symptom may be bone pain or a fracture that occurs with a slight effort. It is the pain from the metastases to the bone that brings the patient to see the doctor. In many cases there are no symptoms, but the cancer is found by diligent digital examination of the rectum. A good diagnostician will suspect cancer of the prostate by the examination, which reveals an irregular gland as hard as stone.

"The stony prostate is cancer unless proven otherwise." Sometimes the symptoms of prostatic enlargement already described may occur. The diagnosis is confirmed by a needle biopsy of the prostate through the rectum.

INCIDENCE OF THE DISEASE

Cancer of the prostate is the most common cancer found in older men, next to cancer of the skin. This illness is so common that 50 percent of elderly men who are autopsied are found to have cancer in their prostatic gland. This type of cancer is called noninvasive, which is reminiscent of those that are found in cancer of the cervix—in situ in the cervix—already discussed. The cause of this cancer remains a mystery, but its incidence has been epidemiologically described to be higher in people who live in the city rather than the country, and those who have immigrated to the United States.

The benign prostatic enlargement (noncancerous enlargement described before) does not seem to be a premalignant condition.

The disheartening fact is that only 30 percent of new cases are discovered by rectal examination and that 80 percent of cases which have been discovered have already spread. Ten percent of new cancers of the prostate are discovered during the removal of noncancerous prostatic enlargement.

Laboratory Examinations for Cancer of the Prostate

Previously it was thought an enzyme called acid phosphatase found in the blood was diagnostic of cancer of the prostate. Soon it was learned that when this enzyme is found to be elevated in the blood, the disease has already spread from its confinement to other parts of the body. It is usually normal in early cancer of the prostate.

Treatment of Cancer of the Prostate Gland

The controversy over the proper treatment of cancer of the prostate rages among surgeons, cancer specialists, and medical men. In fact, even today controversial treatment is being given, from surgery which is mutilative to radiation and chemical therapy.

The treatment of this malignancy is dependent on the stage of the disease. Staging is necessary in order to develop a nationwide concept of the modality and prognosis of the disease. The folks in California will be able to communicate their results of treatment to the folks in Maine—a uniformity of language and definition is needed.

To simplify the concepts of treatment of cancer of the prostate, we can simply state that two large categories are 1) cancer of the prostate confined to that gland, and 2) cancer of the prostate that has spread to neighboring organs and to distant sites.

The classification below is a refinement of these simplified categories.

CLINICAL STAGES

Stage A: Defined as being unsuspected clinically, as found in routine autopsy examination (pathologist's cancer).

Stage B: Defined as long as two decades ago as a neoplasm that, on digital examination, was totally confined to the prostate. Digital finger examination of the rectum underestimates the extent of the prostatic cancer.

Stage C: Defined as a neoplasm that, on rectal examination, has extended beyond the shell of the prostate gland into the surrounding tissues, but not to distant sites. Forty percent of all new cancers are found at stage C, in contrast to 10 percent in stage B.

Stage D: Patients who have cancer of the prostate with spread to other parts of the body. Unfortunately, many patients in this stage are the first ones found.

HORMONAL TREATMENT

The first form of treatment given for cancer, hormonal treatment, was welcomed with exhilaration and optimism. In some cases this has been justified; for example, cancer of the ovaries sometimes improves with a female hormone. Such was the triumphant exclamation of the treatment of prostatic cancer in 1941. Charles B. Huggins demonstrated that castration or the administration of female hormones could cause the regression of cancer of the prostate and its spread. Then we soon learned that there were some cancers of the prostate that did not respond; others became resistant, some did not respond at all. Furthermore, after a long period of treatment, the majority failed to respond.

It became commonplace to treat cancers of the prostate, whether they had spread or not, with female hormones. Female hormones—making men's breasts enlarge, causing them to be impotent, and even inducing cardiovascular accidents such as heart attacks, strokes, and embolism as the results of a tendency to clot—did not stop the hormone enthusiasts. Today we know those patients who were given estrogens derived no benefit from their anticancer effect because so many men died from heart attacks rather than their illness.

SURGICAL TREATMENT

Early in the fifties radical surgery was considered the form of treatment of prostatic cancer. This operation is a destructive procedure, which removes the prostate, the tissues, and the lymph glands; leaves the patient impotent, sometimes incontinent (no control over urination); and does not cure the patient any more than the hormonal treatment did. Today there are still urologists who perform this operation and a second opinion is indicated. This operation not only causes the effects mentioned, but, as this operation is radical, its complications are also vast.

TREATMENT ACCORDING TO STAGE

In stage A disease (asymptomatic prostatic cancer, sometimes called the pathologist's cancer), radical prostatectomy should not be performed, and, above all, endocrine therapy should not be used. In the early stage the majority of urologists feel that no treatment at all should be given, but careful follow-up by adequate digital annual rectal examination be done. If the patient has symptoms of mild urinary tract obstruction, a much simpler operation, a transurethral resection, through the penis can be performed. Removal of the testicles, called *orchiectomy,* is not indicated under any circumstances, as estrogen therapy (female hormones) is as effective as the removal of the testicles. If estrogen therapy is contemplated and the side effects explained to the patient, then castration can be avoided.

Stage B cancer of the prostate is confined to the gland and is the stage the urologist hopes to find in most patients, or stage A. Unfortunately only 10 percent of stage B carcinomas are found. Stage B cancer of the prostate gland, diagnosed by digital examination, biopsy, and negative evidence of cancer elsewhere, is treated with prostatectomy or radiation.

There is ample evidence now that radiation therapy is as effective as surgery in controlling the local cancer. The patient succumbs from the spread of the cancer of the prostate and not from his local illness. In this situation, before radical surgery is performed, a second opinion should be sought.

Radiation can be given externally or internally. Internal radiation, or implantation of radium, is a surgical procedure that requires general anesthesia, a surgeon, and a radiotherapist. The procedure can last anywhere from two to three hours. External radiation is favored when general anesthesia is a risk, as in patients with heart or lung disease.

We favor implanting radium into the prostate to give a high dosage to this area. Some urologists favor radiation therapy of the entire local area, but side effects, like irritation of the bladder and uncontrollable urgency of urination, irritation of the rectum, and impotence, which occurs in 25 percent of the cases, are unacceptable to many. Implanting local radiation seeds into the prostate has been found to be just as effective and less harmful to the patient.

Stage C carcinoma of the prostate is a cancer that on rectal examination has now gone beyond the capsule into the surrounding tissue. Forty percent of all cancers are found in stage C. Initial treatment for this stage was endocrine manipulations, estrogens, and removal of the testicles. Untreated stage C has an average survival of two to three years. Endocrine manipulation has no effect on cancer survival rates, does not prevent the spread of the cancer, and increases risk of death from heart disease in patients who are treated with estrogens (endocrine therapy). Inserting local radiation has been found to be effective, although radical prostatectomy has also been proven to be theoretically sound. Survival time seems to be the same, whether radical prostatectomy or radiation insertion is done.

Stage D cancer is cancer that has spread to other parts of the body. Estrogen therapy, or hormonal therapy, is indicated for the cancer that has spread to other parts of the body, such as bone, if symptoms are present. Asymptomatic spread of cancer of the prostate requires no treatment. Patients can live long periods of time without treatment and survive well into the eighth decade.

Eighty percent of patients experience improvement when first treated. It has been reported that survival rate with hormonal manipulation in stage D cancer has improved from 6 percent to 40 percent. Unfortunately, in spite of excellent response, in stage D cancer, even with hormonal treatment, symptoms reappear within a year or two, and if they reappear, survival time is only six months in 50 percent of patients. If there are no signs of obstruction from the prostate, prostatectomy is generally not performed if the cancer has spread, but extended radiation therapy is used along with hormonal therapy.

We do not favor the removal of other glands, as the adrenals and the pituitary, for metastases of cancer of the prostate.

If the spread of the tumor is not responsive to hormonal treatments, chemotherapy is presently used with some success.

The prevention of cancer of the prostate would be screening for asymptomatic patients with potentially curable lesions, relying primarily upon an intelligent, experienced finger. A physical examination must include a rectal examination.

7: Cancer of the Bladder

IN VICTORIAN ENGLAND it was fashionable for the middle and upper classes to have their chimneys cleaned by eight-year-old urchins. These youngsters, undernourished, slight in stature, were lowered through the chimney by their masters to clean the passageways. The life span of these enslaved children was generally short, as they died from pulmonary complications and cancer of the bladder and rectum. Other occupations responsible for bladder cancer were found in 1900 in workers of aniline dye factories of the German empire. A sickly pun at that time was that "dye workers die." The Germans studied these cases and found that the length of dye exposure varied considerably and the chemical agent was recognized as beta naphthylamine diphenyl. These same aniline dye factories later were easily converted to ammunition production during the First and Second World Wars.

Another associated cause of bladder cancers is cigarette smoking. Throughout this book cigarette smoking is implicated in many diseases such as lung cancer, arteriosclerosis, strokes, heart attacks, and cancer of the bladder because of the tar contained in the smoke. Bladder stones, chronic parasitic infections of the type found in Egypt, called schistosoma, are also associated with malignancy.

The Incidence of the Disease

There are thirty thousand cases estimated each year, with approximately ten thousand dying in the same period. One of the recent publicized deaths was Hubert Humphrey.

Symptoms of Cancer of the Bladder

This is a disease that remains localized for a long period of time within the bladder wall. During a period of latency there is no evidence of the neoplasm. Later, as the cancer grows, clinical evidence becomes apparent. This cancer spreads through lymph nodes to bone, lung, liver, and to all parts of the body through the blood and lymph glands.

The most common symptom in a patient with bladder cancer is blood in the urine, called *hematuria*. Patients who have the earliest form of cancer, called cancer in situ, may occasionally complain of difficulty in urination, burning, and frequency, not unlike the symptoms seen with the prostate disease.

Diagnosis of Cancer of the Bladder

By studying the cells from the urinary bladder, called *urinary cytology*, early cancer sometimes can be diagnosed. The more advanced the cancer, the more readily are these bladder-washing cells positive. By studying the urine for bladder-wall cells with techniques similar to pap smear, early cancer sometimes can be diagnosed. The more advanced the cancer, the more readily are these bladder washings positive. Cystoscopy, which we have already described, with biopsy is used for the diagnosis.

Treatment of Cancer of the Bladder

This is a controversial issue. If the tumor is merely a finger-like growth of tissue, called a *papilloma*, it can be removed through the penis, using a cystoscope, with a complete cure. Regrowth, however, is not uncommon. This is not a cancerous lesion. If the tumor cannot be removed in this way (see prostate chapter), part of the bladder containing the tumor can be resected.

If there is frank cancer, more radical surgery consists of the entire removal of the bladder, called *cystectomy*. The urine is diverted through a small piece of intestine that is connected to the abdominal wall. Now the urine is collected by a plastic bag.

The major controversy occurs when the tumor has progressed to a stage beyond the bladder, and concerns whether the combination of radiation and surgery should be used. Some reports indicate that preoperative radiation followed by complete removal of the tumor gives the same survival rate as operation without radiation. Radiation alone seems to be inadequate as compared with radiation with radical removal of the bladder.

This tumor is also of interest in that some patients have a natural immunity to it; there are, as a matter of fact, cells called *lymphocytes,* which actually destroy the tumor without any treatment. The host may destroy the neoplasm, which accounts for the miraculous cure of bladder tumors without treatment.

Cause of This Finding

The overall five-year survival rate for cancer of the bladder appears to be in the vicinity of 62 percent. Although saccharin has been implicated in cancer of the bladder, it has not been proven to be causative, while cyclamates have a very strong relationship between their chronic use and bladder cancer.

The elimination of carcinogens—especially cigarette smoking—and chronic infections may hold the key for the control of this cancer.

8: Surgery for Impotence

IMPOTENCE MEANS the inability to initiate or maintain an erection; it is not synonymous with loss of sexual desire. There are almost ten to fifteen million males affected with this humiliating condition, from ages eighteen to eighty. Most males at some time in their lives suffer from this ignoble state, usually on a temporary basis, but too many times it becomes a chronic disability.

The cause of impotence can be from psychiatric or physical problems, such as diabetes, cancer, or circulatory disorders. Common psychiatric reasons are chronic depression and anxiety. Cure is often possible once depression is identified as a cause.

Numerous medications can cause impotence, from the common varieties of drugs used to treat hypertension and heart disease to some popular tranquillizers. Alcohol, by far, is the most common orally taken substance associated with a high degree of impotence. William Shakespeare well understood how alcohol interferes with sexual functions. A quote from *Macbeth*, Act II, Scene 3, illustrates this:

MACDUFF: What three things does drink especially provoke?
PORTER: Merry, sir, nose-painting, sleep, and urine. Lechery, sir, it provokes, and unprovokes: it provokes the desire, but it takes away the performance.

Historically and to the present day, impotence erroneously is identified with loss of masculinity and strength. In biblical times a king's power was directly linked to fertility and potency. When King David's erections were not restored by fair young virgins, he stepped down from the throne in favor of Adonijah.

Some physicians feel that impotence has increased in our generation and claim it is actually in epidemic form, striking the very young as well as the middle-aged person. The problem of impotence has been a subject of humorous anecdotes but is no laughing matter. Impotence is included in this book, as there are surgical measures to help correct this dreadful universal problem. Before rushing to have surgical correction, a second opinion is necessary. This form of treatment is still too new to receive universal acceptance, and is receiving too much unwarranted publicity.

Medical treatment, for the most part, has been unsuccessful, although there has been recent interest in psychiatric sexual training and education as championed by Masters and Johnson. Attempts to treat impotence by the use of aphrodisiacs have primarily a placebo effect. An entire manuscript could be spent on the different forms that have been used: food, drugs, and drinks have been advocated to stimulate a sexual desire and power with little justification. Simple substances, such as red-hot pepper, hard-boiled eggs, to more sophisticated methods, such as cannabis, strychnine, ergot, vitamin E, vitamin C, ginseng, catharsis with nux vomica, iron, cold douches to the perineum, tonics, gold, and sodium have been advocated. Today, in the Far East, concoctions consisting of calf's testicles blended with brandy hold favor. Unfortunately male hormones are commonly given, generally with little success; as a matter of fact, they may actually suppress the body's ability to form the male hormone and thus compound the problem.

When impotence is not due to psychiatric causes, surgical treatment may be indicated. This treatment is four centuries old. At the present time surgical treatment of impotence consists of implantation of an inflatable cylinder into the wall of the penis. Some of the earlier devices were not inflatable, but gave a permanent erection to the patient.

The device is simple enough. The patient activates it by repeatedly squeezing the bulb pump in the scrotum to pump fluid from the reservoir which is underneath the abdominal muscle into cylinders implanted inside the penis. A pressure of 200 cm of water usually makes the penis sufficiently rigid for intercourse. After intercourse the patient activates a release valve in the pump by pushing a button for a few seconds. The fluid then moves back into the reservoir and the penis again becomes limp.

Prior to an operation, a thorough medical diagnostic workup should be done on the patient, along with a psychiatrist, before the decision is made for the implant. Patients who received the implant vary from the age of twenty-one to eighty-five. Most of the patients who have had the operation had diabetes or other physical illnesses.

There are too few patients who have had this procedure to make a valid evaluation; however, a recent study in New York, where thirty-one wives of men who received the implant were interviewed, is worth reviewing. It was pointed out there were men who have not used them at all months after surgery, and there were wives who did not know until the surgery that the implant had been done. Most women complained that the implant was too hard and painful, that it buckled and bent, that extra lubrication needed to be used; others have complained that the implant was too large.

Surgeons state that the device can last twenty years. Manufacturers sell the device to hospitals and then the hospitals sell it to surgeons qualified to implant it. The manufacturer maintains a list of trained surgeons.

Men with psychogenic impotence who were refractory to all forms of treatment have received the prosthesis.

Before the male decides to undergo this operation, careful understanding and discussion with his sexual partner is indicated. An exhaustive search for the medical or psychiatric cause of the impotence needs to be carried out. Treatment by a competent sex therapist should be attempted. Then, if everything else fails, surgery can be considered. A surgeon who has experience with this procedure must be found in order to assure some degree of success.

9: Vascular Surgery

ARTERIOSCLEROSIS: DISEASE OF THE ARTERIES

Historical Aspects

THE HISTORY OF VASCULAR SURGERY dates back to the early time when physicians were concerned with the control of massive hemorrhage. Galen, then a newly trained doctor, was employed by the Roman emperor to be the physician of the gladiators. In this role it was he who made keen observations on bleeding arteries and ligation of bleeding vessels. It was rumored throughout Rome that he carried a beating heart from the Forum to study its function. As happened with many advanced techniques from those enlightened times, they were lost during the Middle Ages. Cautery with branding iron or boiling oil became the accepted methods of hemorrhage control.

In 1564 the great French military surgeon, Ambroise Paré, introduced ligation of blood vessels. It was not until late in the eighteenth century that any attempt was made to repair injured blood vessels. In 1830 George James Guthrie, an English surgeon, accomplished the first successful repair of a vein. In the early part of the twentieth century Alexis Carrel, the French surgeon and Nobel Prize winner in physiology and medicine, developed new techniques for suturing blood vessels. His work remained unappreciated and forgotten until the 1940s, following the discovery of heparin, which allowed surgeons to prevent blood clotting while operating on temporarily occluded arteries.

Work on artificial arteries was initiated by Dr. Robert Gross. Since that time further research has developed artificial grafts. Early in the modern development of vascular surgery it was learned that the patient's own vein, when available, is the best material for creating an artificial artery.

Surgical techniques for the repair and replacement of diseased arteries developed following the Second World War. Large numbers of operations are now done throughout the world to restore inadequate blood flow to the lower portion of the body and legs, or to replace or repair extensively diseased arteries. In the United States, in particular, with the ever-increasing age of the population, these techniques are receiving widespread application.

Prevalence of Arteriosclerosis

Arteriosclerosis is the most prevalent disorder of mankind. This disease is an epidemic in affluent nations except Japan, and affects both sexes and all ages, except infants. Clinics across the nation find the number of patients seeking attention for vascular problems is increasing. More diagnostic evaluation is being done with X-ray and non–X-ray techniques than ever before. These patients are hospitalized for longer-than-average hospital stays because of their advanced age and the complex nature of their problems.

Anatomy of Blood Vessels

The main blood vessel in the body is referred to as the aorta. It arises from the left side of the heart, and, at the upper part of the chest, turns toward the back and then descends down the back to the left side of the vertebral column to the level of the belly button. At that level it divides into the main branches to supply each leg.

The wall of arteries is divided into three layers. The outside layer is a loose, fibrous woven matrix referred to as the *adventitia*. The middle layer, which makes up the bulk of the walls, is composed of smooth muscle and elastic tissue. This is an expansile layer which can also contract. It is referred to as the *media*. The inside lining of the artery is referred to as the *intima*. It is a smooth, very flat-celled lining and is supported by a base of loose fibrous strands.

Hardening of the Arteries: Arteriosclerosis

Arteriosclerosis is characterized by the formation of fatty deposits in the intima of the blood vessel. Cholesterol is deposited in this layer. Initially, fatty streaks of the cholesterol are seen in the main blood vessel (aorta) of young children. In industrialized countries, like the United States and Western Europe, these streaks form the primary basis for the development of arteriosclerosis. By the time the young male reaches sixteen to eighteen years, the deposition may have progressed significantly and cholesterol deposits can be seen scattered through the arterial tree. The deposits may enlarge, narrowing the diameter of the passageway where blood is transported.

As the walls become thicker and the cholesterol deposition progresses, the inside lining of the artery is pushed together, obliterating the passageway for carrying blood. This results in the complete blockage of the artery. Before the complete blockage occurs, occasionally the inside lining of the artery becomes disrupted or ulcerated, allowing some of the cholesterol to break off and travel in the bloodstream to other parts of the body, or to become a site of blood-clot formation. In some patients the resultant destruction of the elastic and muscular elements of the middle layer of the blood vessel results in weakening of the arterial walls. Segmental massive dilatation of the artery with very thin, weak walls may be the end result. This ballooned-out area is referred to as an *aneurysm*.

Risk Factors: Development of Arteriosclerosis

Four primary risk factors have been identified. These are 1) cigarette smoking, 2) increased blood pressure, 3) elevated blood-sugar levels (diabetes mellitus), and 4) abnormally high fats circulating in the bloodstream.

EFFECTS OF CIGARETTE SMOKING

A clear measurable effect of cigarette smoking is a decrease in the flow of blood to the fingers and toes. This is because of the effect of nicotine on the small blood vessels. High school students demonstrate this in their laboratories by applying nicotine to the web space on the foot of a frog. With low-power magnification they observe that normal flow through the tiny vessels of the web space abruptly stops and the blood vessels go into spasm. Additionally, cigarette smoking increases the level of circulating blood fats and also affects blood-clotting properties. A study of 401 men with arteriosclerosis who did not have diabetes and were less than sixty years of age revealed that only 2.5 percent were nonsmokers. Patients with arteriosclerosis who are now seen in the authors' offices are first advised to stop smoking before there is any discussion of diet or exercise. Indeed, many vascular surgeons will not consider surgery if the patient continues to smoke.

HYPERTENSION (INCREASED BLOOD PRESSURE)

Studies have demonstrated that hypertension increases the risk of a significant arteriosclerosis in the coronary arteries and in the arteries throughout the body. In fact, at one time it was felt that high blood pressure was the cause of arteriosclerosis. Proper control of elevated blood pressure with medication is essential.

DIABETES MELLITUS (INCREASED BLOOD SUGAR)

Diabetes mellitus is associated with arteriosclerosis at two to three times the incidence of the nondiabetic population. Twenty percent of patients having narrowing or blockage of arteries to the legs due to arteriosclerosis have diabetes mellitus. The inability of the body to properly metabolize carbohydrates is linked with the deposition of cholesterol and other fat in the walls of arteries.

CIRCULATING FAT

More than 40 percent of the adult population in the United States is 20 pounds overweight; 40 percent of the daily caloric intake of adults is in the form of saturated fats. Circulating cholesterol levels are at least partially related to the ingestion of fat. Dietary changes can control the cholesterol levels of most patients; abstinence from cigarettes will make that control far easier. Some patients with elevated cholesterol levels are not responsive to dietary management. Such patients do carry an increased risk of hardening of the arteries, as is true of most of their family members.

Exciting new research has demonstrated that fat travels in two forms in the bloodstream. These are referred to as *high-density* and *low-density lipoproteins* (HDL and LDL). Blood tests can be done to demonstrate these levels in an individual. The HDL level seems to bind the cholesterol so that it cannot be deposited in the arteries. Exercise and moderate alcohol intake have been demonstrated to increase the HDL level. High HDL levels are associated with minimal risk of coronary artery disease.

Carotid Artery Disease

The carotid arteries supply the face and the brain with blood. These arteries arise out of the chest in the base of the neck and travel on its left and right sides.

Arteriosclerosis of the carotid artery can cause narrowing with reduced flow to the brain. The patient, usually in the fifth decade of life or older, may complain of the temporary loss of speech or inability to move an arm or a leg. The symptoms are transient, lasting less than an hour. Called TIAs (transient ischemic attacks—the type Presidents Woodrow Wilson and Franklin D. Roosevelt allegedly suffered), they are due to decreased blood flow to the brain. On examination a murmur, technically called a *bruit,* is heard at the angle of the jaw where the main carotid artery branches.

The usual cause is a piece of cholesterol from an ulcerated area in the carotid artery breaking off and traveling in the bloodstream to a small blood vessel of the brain, temporarily shutting down its blood supply. The patient is in danger of experiencing a stroke, resulting in permanent damage.

Evaluation of a Patient

Once the clinical diagnosis of arterial disease is made, further diagnostic studies are in order.

The most complete technique is an X-ray procedure designed to obtain a road map of the condition of the arteries: *arteriography.* Dye is injected directly into the arteries and can display aneurysms, ulcers, or blockages of vessels.

Arteriography requires a needle puncture of an artery and a long tube, which is passed into the artery under fluoroscopy, followed by the injection of the dye. Anytime an artery is punctured, there is a risk of possible hemorrhage or thrombosis at the puncture site. This is extremely uncommon, a risk not greater than 1 percent. It is impossible to consider patients seriously for vascular surgery without proper arteriography.

There are other techniques for evaluating arterial problems

that do not involve a needle puncture of an artery and are therefore considered noninvasive. These are relatively new techniques for measuring flow and direction of flow with sonar-like and volume-recording instruments. They are helpful only in that they may indicate the presence or absence of significant problems but do not eliminate the need for arteriography.

TREATMENT

Surgeons and internists do not agree on the management of these patients. Surgeons feel strongly that if such patients have normal tests such as brain wave (electroencephalogram), skull X rays, and a brain scan, they should then have X rays of the arteries to the brain. The surgeon is looking for an area of marked narrowing—greater than 80 percent. He is also looking for an area that may demonstrate a clear "ulcer pocket." Such findings can be corrected by surgery.

Aspirin has been shown to affect the sticky portion of the blood, called *platelets*. Platelets are derived from special cells and initiate blood clotting. When an ulcer forms in an artery, or when a blood vessel is injured, the artery produces a chemical substance that stimulates the platelets to agglutinate in the damaged area, thereby triggering the entire mechanism for blood-clot formation. If patients with carotid artery ulcers are given aspirin, there is a good chance that a clot will not form. Surgeons point out that an ulcer is dangerous, not only because of the blood clot, but because the cholesterol itself travels in the bloodstream up to the brain. There is no protection from aspirin for this problem. If an arteriogram proves that a severe stenosis or an ulcer is present, surgery is straightforward, safe, and curative.

THE MEDICAL OPINION OF TRANSIENT ISCHEMIC ATTACKS RESULTING FROM CAROTID ARTERY DISEASE (LITTLE STROKES AND THE PREVENTION OF STROKES)

In order to determine the benefits and risks of any form of treatment, one must be aware of the natural history of the disease process. From a study at the Mayo Clinic, the following facts came forth. Among patients with little strokes who do not die of a cause other than the stroke, about one-third will suffer a stroke within five years of the first attack. Patients who have had transient ischemic attacks will experience a stroke within five years; more than 20 percent will do so within one month of the initial attack, and 50 percent will do so within one year. Many patients only have a single attack before suffering a stroke. Patients with a high-grade obstruction of the carotid artery have a greater stroke risk than patients with minimal stenosis.

The conclusion of the Mayo Clinic's studies are:

1. The greatest risk of strokes occurs in the first year following the onset of the transient ischemic attack, especially the first two months.

2. No study has shown that any single mode of treatment of this condition, either surgical or medical, is superior for preventing a stroke.

3. In experienced hands carotid surgery is a safe procedure that can effectively reduce the symptoms and may lower the risk of a stroke in some selective patients.

4. Anticoagulant treatment does not appear to affect survival rate after the onset of transient ischemic attacks. This anticoagulant treatment increases the risk of hemorrhage when used for one year or more.

It appears that aspirin decreases the risk of stroke in men, but not in women. The medical opinion is that aspirin prevents the attack but does not prolong the life of the patient. The majority of patients with transient ischemic attacks die from myocardial infarction, whether they receive the surgical treatment or the medical treatment.

There may be several mechanisms that cause transient ischemic attacks. Fifty percent of those experiencing these attacks show some narrowing or occlusions of the artery, which are surgically accessible. A large group of patients has the same symptoms with no evidence of occlusion of the arteries, and there are numerous asymptomatic patients whose arteriograms revealed arteriosclerosis. In those patients who have no symptoms, the medical man prefers using aspirin to prevent any future transient ischemic attacks, rather than surgery.

Cessation of cigarette smoking, control of hypertension and diabetes, and weight reduction make up part of the essential elements for the reduction of stroke. As a point of fact, strokes have been reduced by 20 percent in the past ten years. There are some studies that seem to indicate that, by drastic reduction of the fat content of the blood by dietary means and medication, some of the arteriosclerotic plaques are reversible.

In a clearly defined case of a transient ischemic attack with excellent arteriographic evidence that an ulcerated plaque is present and with the availability of a surgeon who has performed this operation frequently, the authors would consider surgery in selective cases. It is, however, essential that a proper clinical assessment be made before an arteriogram or surgery is performed. Dizziness and light-headedness are common in the elderly but do not necessarily imply vascular inadequacy to the brain. Generalized numbness, fatigue, blurred vision, weakness, and instability of walk are common complaints which do not necessarily mean impaired blood flow to the brain. The presence of a bruit in the neck, unless it can be correlated with symptoms, has no significance other than presumption that the patient has stenosis of his arteries.

Aneurysms

An abdominal aneurysm is a life-threatening deformity of blood vessels. It represents a weak area of the artery that has ballooned out and is in danger of rupturing, resulting in bleeding into the abdominal cavity or into the muscles of the back. The patient with an aneurysm may suddenly complain of severe abdominal pain. If the patient with this pain is bleeding into his abdominal cavity, he may not survive the trip to the hospital emergency room.

An asymptomatic aneurysm found at routine examination must be thoroughly investigated by the physician. An excellent method of diagnosing an abdominal aneurysm is through ultrasound; the sound-wave technique enables the physician to judge the size of the aneurysm and to recommend surgery when a critical size has been reached.

Should the aneurysm prove to be greater than 4.5 cm in diameter, elective surgery to replace it with a woven Dacron graft is indicated. The risk of sudden, unpredictable rupture is a life-threatening complication carrying a mortality rate of 40 percent. Elective surgery carries a mortality rate of less than 5 percent. The only justification for not recommending surgery is if the patient has severe heart disease, lung disease, kidney disease, or has had a previous stroke or is senile.

SOME HISTORICAL NOTATIONS ON THE HISTORY OF ANEURYSM

Attempts at ligation of aneurysm date back to the 1700s. The Italian surgeon, Giovanni Maria Lancisi, physician to the pope, often regarded as the founder of cardiology, wrote a dissertation on aneurysm which was published in 1728. He told the story of a man, fifty-five years old, fond of singing, who harbored a large aortic aneurysm protruding from his chest. Lancisi advised him to refrain from exertion, including singing, which could cause rupture of the aneurysm. The patient asked a famous local surgeon of the day to provide a device to wear around his chest to restrain the thrust of the bulging aneurysm and prevent it from breaking. The surgeon made an iron belt with a spring, not unlike the spring truss worn by a patient with a hernia to retain the protrusion within the thorax. With this belt he kept the aneurysm within the chest. The patient continued to sing merrily until he suddenly died. Operations for aneurysms have been repeated numerous times, but, until recently, they universally failed. In fact, the actual successful operation of the aorta for aneurysm was seen only in 1950 with a proper resection and placement of a graft.

The medical man fully agrees and applauds the surgeon's excellent management of abdominal aneurysms, as this is a preventable cause of sudden death; the medical man encourages other physicians to use techniques such as ultrasonography to diagnose asymptomatic abdominal aneurysms, which need to be repaired before a catastrophe occurs. Too often this diagnosis is completely missed by the practicing physician, either because he does not feel the pulsating mass through the abdomen, or he does not think of it when symptoms like back pain arise. Too often in the emergency room this diagnosis is missed, when a patient who arrives in shock is assumed to have had a heart attack and not a ruptured abdominal aneurysm.

Routine chest X rays are done to find abnormalities of the heart and lung. Ultrasonography of the abdomen is safe and accurate and perhaps should be used as a part of a routine examination in high-risk patients: patients who have hypertension, diabetes, are heavy smokers, and have a family history of arteriosclerosis.

Peripheral Vascular Disease
(Arteriosclerosis of the Arteries of the Leg)

ANATOMY

When arteries of the leg become impacted with the arteriosclerotic material and the flow through them diminishes, sometimes to a mere trickle, this condition is known as peripheral vascular disease.

SYMPTOMS

The earliest symptom of this affliction is pain in the calf after walking a certain distance. When the patient stops walking, the pain subsides. As the disease progresses (and it may not), the distance that the patient can walk becomes shorter and shorter. The feet become cold, especially at night, and develop a reddish-purple discoloration accompanied with tingling sensations. If further progression occurs, gangrene of the toes can develop.

DIAGNOSIS

The physician's examination will reveal cold extremities and decreased or absent pulses in the lower legs. The finding can then be confirmed with an X-ray examination (arteriography) and a sound-wave apparatus called a Doppler, which echoes the state of circulation through the arteries of the legs.

TREATMENT

The surgery performed for this problem is a bypass graft. The long vein is taken from the same leg, properly cleansed, and sewn in place above and below the blockage. It functions as an artery when this procedure is meticulously done. Not all patients, however, can have this type of bypass surgery; it depends on the extent of their disease. There must be a good vessel in the lower leg to sew the graft into which will accommodate the rush of blood. If there are not adequate vessels below the level of the blockage, then the foot may be doomed and amputation may be the ultimate solution.

THE MEDICAL POINT OF VIEW OF PERIPHERAL VASCULAR DISEASE

Before deciding on surgery, a patient needs a thorough trial of medical management, especially if the patient is of an advanced age. Cessation of cigarette smoking is mandatory as well as control of hypertension, diabetes, excess fat in the blood, and overweight (obesity).

One of the outstanding measures is the protection of the poor circulation in the limbs. Half of the patients who undergo amputations as a result of this illness do so because of trauma or mechanical or thermal injury. Many limbs can be saved if the patient is careful not to injure or burn himself, as ulceration of the legs may follow, making salvage difficult.

Measures to improve the circulation have been of little benefit. In the past, measures such as typhoid vaccine have been used to cause a high fever and vasodilatation, with temporary relief of pain and ulcers. Use of vasodilator drugs sometimes increases the blood flow to the skin and muscles, but it seems to be of little help in the control of pain. In the event that there is a sudden acute occlusion of an artery, surgery must be performed swiftly, as in the case of a clot that has traveled from the heart to the leg after a heart attack, causing severe and excruciating pain in the limb. The clot must be swiftly removed; otherwise the limb will be lost.

Many patients tolerate this pain (called intermittent claudication) and require no treatment, especially if there is no evidence of progression of the disease. If the symptoms increase and life becomes intolerable, then surgery is needed. Progression of this illness, in many cases, is halted or slowed by cessation of smoking.

VARICOSE VEINS

When veins in the legs become tortuous and swollen, like a bag of worms, we speak of *varicose veins* or *varicosities.* Known since the time of Hippocrates for their unappetizing appearance, and at times their serious consequences, they can be treated surgically and medically, and another controversy comes to bear.

Incidence of the Illness and Symptoms

One in five American women and one in fifteen men suffer from these swollen veins. Many are aware of a nagging discomfort in their legs with a feeling of fatigue, especially toward the end of the day.

Anatomy of Varicose Vein Formation

The veins carry blood back to the heart, and the arteries carry blood away from the heart. By means of one-way valves, the veins keep the blood flowing toward the heart with the assistance of muscle contractions. If these valves fail, blood will accumulate in the veins and the bulging begins. Pregnancy, straining at stool, obesity can cause this condition to sppear and worsen preexisting varicosities.

These distended veins can develop clots and become inflamed from a variety of causes, like prolonged sitting or crossing of legs, or slight injuries to the legs. This is called superficial phlebitis; it is a painful nuisance but not dangerous. In contradistinction to this is deep thrombophlebitis, a dangerous condition because the clot that is localized deep in the venous system can dislodge and travel to the lung. This is known as an embolism; it is a medical emergency.

Sometimes the varices can start to bleed spontaneously or from a minor injury. This is not a serious problem and can be handled easily by lying down, elevating the leg, and placing gentle pressure at the site of bleeding.

Treatment of Varicose Veins: The Surgeon's View

Most patients go through their entire lives with their varicosities with no mishaps. The major reason to perform surgery is for cosmetic purposes.

Spidery, blue-red vessels of the skin that look like a road map are not varicose veins, but simple dilatations of superficial small veins. Treatment of this condition is not surgery but injections with chemicals to improve their appearance.

One of the dreaded complications of varicose veins is the varicose ulcer. Generally, the seat of this lesion is located on the lower portion of the leg where the circulation is the poorest and trauma is the easiest. A slight bang on the leg from a chair, a bicycle, or any blunt instrument can cause the skin slowly to break down with the formation of an ulcer. If this ulcer is not treated properly, it can become chronic and enlarge to such an extent that only skin grafting can cure it. In its severe form prolonged bed rest is necessary with elevation, cleansing, and applications. This problem has been present for thousands of years and a quote from a Greek physician is appropriate:

> Next comes a plump woman, with bad varicose veins and a typical complication thereof, a stubborn ulcer on the ankle which is bandaged. The iatros (Greek physician) begins by taking a pot from the burner and pouring some water first over his hands to check the temperature, then over the woman's hands because the patient would decide whether it was comfortable. The bandages are removed while the ankle is showered with the warm water. It will keep the sore relaxed, thereby preventing spasms. As for the woman's bulging varicose veins, they will remain untouched. As circumstances may indicate puncturing them once in a while, large sores may follow. Now the ankle is sponged with hot vinegar very carefully because the smell of vinegar is supposed to be harmful especially for women. For obstinate ulcers sweet wine in a lot of patients should be enough. A pad of wool dipped in a drug for fresh wounds consisting of dull nuts, vine flowers, alum, and lead oxide, copper oxide, copper acetate, equal parts diluted in water.

Today the present-day varicose ulcers require intense treatment and, many times, hospitalization. This is one of the fundamental reasons for the operation to be performed on a varicosity.

The Medical Treatment of Varicose Veins

Most of the time there is no treatment necessary for varicose veins except for the prevention of such complications as hemorrhages and ulcerations and, commonly, superficial phlebitis.

The prevention of varicose veins is not possible; however, its progression can be halted. Elastic support in the form of stockings or bandages is useful to assist the venous return by collapsing the venous pools and the superficial veins, enhancing efficiency of the pumping action through the compression of calf muscles. Superb elastic stockings, which are made in the United States and Switzerland, provide support for the fragile skin and protection from external trauma. Whenever possible, periodic elevation of the extremities is as important as elastic support in reducing the pressure. Sleeping at night with the foot of the bed elevated helps to empty the veins and prevent the stasis problem. Walking is an excellent form of treatment for varicosity as well as exercises such as jogging, bicycling, and swimming. These exercises help the normal function of the pumping against gravity forces. Walking actually lowers the venous pressure to about one-third of the standing pressure under normal conditions.

Surgery should be performed only if the patient desires a better-looking leg or if the varicosities become periodically infected, thrombosed, and bleed, and there is a danger of ulceration.

The prevention of phlebitis consists of elastic stockings, leg elevation, avoidance of crossing of legs, or prolonged car or plane rides. If long trips are contemplated, then periodic standing and walking about is helpful.

Injection of the venous system, called *sclerotherapy,* is becoming popular in this country. The English have been doing this procedure far longer than we in the United States. A repeated course of injections may be needed, as this treatment is not a permanent cure. It was once popular at the Mayo Clinic in the 1930s, but abandoned because of the high failure rate. Renewed interest in this treatment stems from more effective chemicals used for injections.

Hemorrhoids

Varicose veins involving the anus are called hemorrhoids. Known since Hippocrates' time, these vascular protrusions sometimes become troublesome.

Occurring because of pregnancy, straining at stool, prostate trouble, or for unknown reasons, they make their unwelcomed appearance. The first sign may be a drop of blood in the bowel, which is enough to frighten anyone, or pain and itching may be the outstanding symptoms. The pain may become so severe when the varicose veins become clotted (thrombosed) that the patient walks like a cowboy after a long ride across the prairie.

TREATMENT OF HEMORRHOIDS

Usually hemorrhoids can be managed by nonsurgical means. Keeping the bowels comfortable, taking warm sitz baths, and using local applications of suppositories and ointment were the methods Hippocrates prescribed in his clinic at the Isle of Kos. These methods are still effectively used today.

If bleeding and recurrent pain become a problem, more aggressive treatment is available. Not used often enough in this country is sclerosing therapy, described under the varicose vein section. The rubber band method is another nonsurgical way to handle these purple devils. A rubber band is placed at the base of the hemorrhoids and left in place until it strangulates and falls off. This method is applicable for internal hemorrhoids. Freezing methods, called *cryosurgery*, are also used. These methods can be done in the office without general anesthesia.

Surgery of hemorrhoids, or hemorrhoidectomy, requires several days of hospitalization with a great deal of discomfort and pain, and the use of a general anesthesia or spinal. Before surgery is suggested, the patient should be aware that there may be other alternatives.

10: Back Surgery (Disc Surgery)

A THIRTY-TWO-YEAR-OLD advertising executive spent his week-ends during the summer gardening and playing tennis. On this particular bright spring morning, as he picked up the hundred-pound bag of peat moss, he suddenly felt severe back pain that radiated down his left leg to his toes. He was unable to stand straight, and, even lying flat in bed, the pain was excruciating. His family doctor hospitalized him, and in spite of rest and painkillers, he did not improve. Special X rays called a myelogram (discussed later) were performed, and disclosed that he had a "pinched nerve." He was operated on and became symptom free.

In another part of the city, an obese forty-five-year-old female had been suffering from back problems for the past ten years, accompanied by other complaints—feeling bloated, with swelling of her legs, flushing of her face, and depression with sleep disturbance. The X-ray examination of the back disclosed some arthritic changes compatible with a disc problem (to be discussed later). After seeing many physicians, she came to a neurosurgeon's office, where myelography was performed which showed that she had some impingement of her nerve. Surgery was performed and this obese lady, after surgery, continued to have the same pain. She went to see other neurosurgeons who did other myelograms and another surgical procedure was performed; she still had back pain.

A seventy-five-year-old woman had suddenly complained of severe back pain radiating down her left leg. The pain was so excruciating that she was hospitalized and consulted a neurosurgeon, who advised a myelogram. The myelogram disclosed a pinched nerve and the surgeon advised an operation. The patient continued to have pain going down her leg from her thighs, and on the morning of surgery her family physician saw a rash going down her leg. The rash was typical for shingles. Surgery was canceled. The treatment of shingles was instituted, and she had no further pain.

These three case histories in effect summarize the problem of disc surgery and chronic back pain. Currently it has been estimated that seven million Americans are being treated by doctors for chronic back pain, and new cases are being added at a rate of almost two million per year. Back pain is considered the most prevalent single medical ailment in the United States.

Lumbar disc disease is a group of conditions that includes a general narrowing of the spinal canal which may be either congenital or acquired secondary to extensive arthritis of the spine. With lumbar disc ailments, there is a herniation of the disc located between two vertebral bodies and then pinching-off of the nerve.

This is another controversial subject: sometimes surgery is performed too soon, too frequently, or too infrequently.

Anatomy and Pathology of Discs

A lumbar disc is the structure located between two vertebral bodies of the spinal cord in the lower part of the back (the lumbar region), which acts as a "cushion" for the vertebral bodies. It is composed of cartilage containing a spongy center (the nucleus pulposus) and a fibrous ring (annulus fibrosus) holding it in place. In a soft, herniated lumbar disc there is weakening of the outer fibrous band that holds the center of the disc. The most common position for herniation of disc material is sideways, causing compression of the lumbar nerve roots, usually a branch of the longest nerve in the body, called the sciatic nerve; this condition enervates the lower extremities.

Symptoms of a Herniated Disc or Lumbar Disc Disease

Herniated discs generally occur in younger people, who are active physically; the symptoms consist primarily of severe back pain with radiation down the lower extremity. Lumbar disc disease, which includes general narrowing of the spinal cord, occurs in older people with degenerative arthritis of the spine. In this instance pain may occur in one or both legs, especially on walking or prolonged standing or sitting.

In both of these conditions the patient experiences great difficulties rising up from a chair, bending down, getting dressed, and invariably awakens in the morning with the inability to get out of bed.

Diagnosis of Lumbar Disc Disease

Clinically the diagnosis is easily made by the history and the physical examination. The major pitfall in the diagnosis of a disc disease is an X-ray examination of the spine. In older patients spinal X rays invariably will reveal some osteoarthritis and narrowing of the disc space; yet the symptoms may not be coming from a pinched nerve. In many instances there is little correlation between the X-ray findings and the patient's clinical symptoms.

The definitive diagnosis of compression of a disc on a nerve is performed with a myelogram.

The Procedure of a Myelogram (Myelography)

The purpose is to visualize the space around the spinal cord to find out if there are any lesions of the spinal cord or associated parts of the nervous system. A spinal tap is performed. The patient lies prone on a myelography table, a local anesthetic is given, and a needle is inserted into the spinal space. A small amount of fluid is withdrawn and a contrast medium is injected. The injection table is tilted.

The procedure may last thirty minutes to one and a half hours, depending on the condition of the patient and the experience of the physician. The lumbar puncture causes some pain and a stinging or sensation of pressure may be felt when the contrast material is injected. The patient may also feel sharp, stabbing pains radiating down his leg. It is a very uncomfortable procedure, as the patient is strapped to a table and experiences a great deal of stiffness. The tilting of the table may make the patient feel nauseated and sweaty, and dizziness may occur. For the first twenty-four hours after the study, the patient needs to lie flat and may complain of headache, nausea, back pain, and a stiff neck. Allergic reaction to the contrast material may occur. There is a small possibility of infection, but as a rule the procedure goes on uneventfully.

When the Procedure Should Be Performed: The Surgical Point of View

To make a firm diagnosis and to decide whether the patient needs surgery, a myelography is indicated. When the neurological examination discloses impairment of nerve function, such as loss of knee- and ankle-jerk reflex, and pain is continuous, nonsurgical treatment should not be continued excessively long if there is to be a good result. Pressure on nerves may lead to irreversible damage.

The Medical Point of View

The indications for myelography and surgery are the same. If there is a strong suspicion of a spinal tumor, then myelography should be done. In the event there is pain that does not improve and there is evidence of neurological injury, such as loss of bladder or bowel control, there is little controversy in doing a myelography followed by surgery. However, two-thirds of patients with lumbar discogenic disease may be adequately managed by conservative measures. A prolonged period of strict bed rest, varying from one to four weeks' duration, accompanied by painkillers and muscle relaxants, must be first tried. After the acute symptoms have passed, a course of physiotherapy with back-strengthening exercises is then employed.

A firm diagnosis can be established without a myelogram by adequate clinical examination, and other diseases affecting the spine, such as cancer, have to be ruled out. When the pain becomes severe and is no longer tolerable, and the patient is almost disabled, then myelography and surgery are favored.

Recently, herniated discs have been diagnosed without a myelography through a computer tomography known as CAT scans. At the present time the reliability and the appropriate role of CAT scanning in evaluating patients with low back pain are still in the process of being evaluated.

In the case of the first patient presented in this chapter—a young man who presented with the classical history of a ruptured disc—in spite of prolonged bed rest and treatment he did not recover and surgery was performed with excellent results.

In the second patient, the obese lady, symptoms undoubtedly were not entirely caused by a herniated disc, but were the result of several causes, one of them psychosomatic in origin, and osteoarthritis was also present.

In the third case, the patient had classical myelographic findings and clinical findings, yet she was suffering from shingles. If the rash had not appeared prior to the operation, a needless operation would have been performed. She illustrates that, even with myelographic findings and clinical findings, the cause of the pain may not necessarily be arising from a ruptured disc.

Results of Surgery

Patients with a single disc herniation have a 95 percent chance of excellent results. By good results the surgeon means relief of pain and return of the individual to gainful employment. Other statistics over a ten- to fifteen-year period have shown 75 percent good results.

Failure cases seem to occur in medical-legal as well as compensation cases, where the disc injury allegedly resulted from an accident. The traumatized patient who plans to go on a rampage of suits to recover damages from an autombile accident or other injury sometimes has myeolography and surgery performed too early.

Other Forms of Treatment

Chiropractic manipulation for the treatment of back ailments must proceed with great caution. If a ruptured disc is present, the patient's illness may be compounded and can lead to complete paralysis. If there is no disc injury and the condition is an unstable back resulting from muscle spasms, massage and chiropractic techniques can be helpful.

Recently, injection of cortisone into the spinal canal has been employed for a three-month treatment to avoid surgery. This form of treatment is too new to evaluate but in the future may reduce the necessity for surgery for this ailment.

11: Surgery for Arthritis

"ARTHRITIS IS A MEAN DISEASE." So begins the poem by the poet, Stephen Vincent Benét, one of the hundreds of thousands who has suffered from rheumatoid arthritis.

Arthritis is the most prevalent disease in the United States. There are twice as many patients suffering from this illness as from heart disease or high blood pressure. This miserable illness costs the nation over $1.5 billion per year in lost wages and $1.2 billion per year in medical costs.

Arthritis is defined as an illness involving the joints and joint structures, and is characterized by pain, swelling, and stiffness. Rheumatism is an affliction of the muscles that support the joints.

The word *arthritis* was used by Hippcrates in 460 B.C. It means inflammation of joints—hot, red, swollen, painful joints. Galen, the Greek physician, in the year A.D. 130, introduced the word *rheumatism*, which means "flux or discharge or mucous of evil humours." It encompassed the theory that all illnesses result from the "humours of the body being off balance."

[154]

There are numerous forms of rheumatic disease, but 75 percent of rheumatic sufferers either have rheumatoid arthritis or osteoarthritis. Arthritis is a prominent feature of at least thirty-five illnesses. For example, gonorrhea can cause arthritis.

Rheumatoid arthritis is a progressive chronic illness that destroys joint tissue and can affect many organs of the body, including the heart, the lungs, and the blood system. Degenerative arthritis afflicts only the joints and as a rule does not have the same crippling impact as rheumatoid arthritis.

The Cause of Rheumatoid Arthritis

The cause of this illness is unknown. Speculations include improper diet, climate, dampness, viruses, and toxic agents, but none of these has been proven to be the cause.

Onset of Rheumatoid Arthritis

This disease afflicts women three times more than men. Eighty percent of cases occur between the ages of twenty-five and forty-five, with a peak incidence between thirty-five and forty. Rheumatoid arthritis occurring in teen-agers or youngsters is called juvenile arthritis.

Diagnosis of Rheumatoid Arthritis

"All joints that hurt ain't rheumatoid arthritis." So goes the saying of rheumatologists. Sometimes in the beginning of the illness it is impossible to make a clear diagnosis because of its nonspecific nature: joint swelling and pain, which may occur in other diseases.

The onset may be sudden, with acute swelling of one or two joints accompanied by redness and pain, or it may be subtle with only some morning stiffness. Generally it may begin with one joint and eventually a second joint is involved, with the smaller joints of the hands particularly affected. The knuckle joints of the fingers are involved as well as the end joints. Accompanying these symptoms is stiffness, especially in the morning, of at least three hours' duration.

The correct diagnosis of rheumatoid arthritis is essential, as the prognosis is different from any other illness. Likewise its treatment needs to be taken on with a vigorous, knowledgeable, trained, experienced approach; otherwise crippling may quickly follow, which, in many instances, can be avoided. Too many patients are treated inadequately from a lack of interest and knowledge.

Course of the Disease

Sometimes the disease is cured spontaneously, never to reappear again. Other times it may disappear and reappear and remain active indefinitely. Traditionally, this is a chronic progressive illness leading to joint deformity, destruction of the cartilage of the joint, subluxations, and final total disability. Pain and stiffness are a constant accompaniment of this illness, coupled with frustrations for the physician and the patient.

Treatment of Rheumatoid Arthritis

Great strides have been made in understanding this malady, along with effective treatment that includes medical and surgical disciplines. Unfortunately, the physician's interest in and knowledge of the treatment is often lacking. The attitude of physicians toward arthritis was well expressed by William Osler, considered the father of modern medicine. He once said, "When I see an arthritic come in the front door, I want to leave by the back door." Doctors who specialize in these illnesses are called rheumatologists. An enthusiastic and optimistic attitude on the part of the physician, coupled with discrete medications and expert physical therapy, can lessen or even prevent deformity.

In the past treatment of rheumatoid arthritis consisted of

every imaginable concoction—from vitamins to diets low in salt, sugar, fat, protein—and all have met with failure. The most outlandish treatment yet described consists of patients being exposed to a minor degree of radioactivity. Old abandoned uranium mines have been converted to arthritic centers. For an exorbitant fee, patients sit on wooden stools for a prescribed period of time, allegedly receiving enough radiation to cure the illness. Rheumatoid patients are seen wearing copper bracelets, electrical bracelets, and special garters. The shelves are stacked with an endless row of pills. Chiropractors and acupuncturers claim to have the answers.

Why all the claims of treatment cures are so readily accepted by the public is not difficult to understand. The treatment dilemma arises because patients with rheumatoid arthritis have spontaneous remissions; some get better no matter what is done. Placebos make some patients feel better. Every new pill that has been marketed by the pharmaceutical companies in recent years has an exhilarating effect when first used by the rheumatoid patient and then loses its effect.

The most reliable form of treatment, which is two thousand years old and is still the mainstay to this day, is aspirin.

Aspirin

Aspirin is derived from the willow and other plants used as medications since antiquity. Hippocrates, two thousand years ago, recommended chewing willow bark for the treatment of childbirth pain. In Rome, Pliny the Elder user a poplar bark for back pain. American Indians made tea from the willow bark to reduce fever, and the Hottentots in Africa prepared a similar brew for rheumatic pains. A German chemist suffering from rheumatism asked his son to devise a form of aspirin that he could tolerate. In 1893 Felix Hoffman came up with the aspirin we know today. It is an effective drug for the treatment of rheumatoid arthritis when used in the correct dosages to arrive at a certain blood level. Aspirin reduces the pain and swelling of joints and eliminates stiffness. Its major drawback is that it sometimes causes serious irritation of the stomach and bleeding.

In the United States the American pharmaceutical industry produces 12,000 tons of aspirin per year for domestic consumption. This is equivalent to 150 aspirin tablets for every man, woman, and child in this country.

If aspirin is not effective, then gold therapy (gold salts) is added. At the present time it is the most effective form of treatment for rheumatoid arthritis, along with aspirin. In many cases it may actually halt the illness or at least keep the patient comfortable throughout his life. Gold must be administered by a physician who is experienced in using this medication, as it occasionally does have side effects.

Other anti-arthritis medications, too numerous to list, in most cases are as effective as aspirin, perhaps a little better.

Cortisone is used too frequently and too indiscriminately for this illness, although symptoms in individual joints can be relieved by injecting cortisone into them. Cortisone given by mouth may have serious side effects, and can actually worsen the disease. Cortisone was first thought to be a "miracle drug" in the 1950s when it was found that pregnant women with rheumatoid arthritis went into remission. It was discovered that the body's own cortisone level in pregnant patients increases and makes the joints improve. Cortisone should be the last resort in medication, as it can cause further destruction of joints and has widespread side effects.

Physical therapy is effective in lessening deformity and improving function and vitality. But in spite of excellent treatment, whether it be aspirin, other anti-inflammatory agents, or gold, in many patients the disease progresses relentlessly with complete destruction of the joints; this is where the surgeon enters the picture.

Hand and Wrist Surgery

The loss of wrist motion is an unfortunate tragedy for the patient with rheumatoid arthritis, causing considerable functional restrictions in eating, personal hygiene, and general daily activities.

Synovectomy, or removal of the capsule (membrane surrounding the joint), provides some relief of pain. Pain is the major indication for performing surgery in rheumatoid arthritis. Cosmetic appearance of the hand is of little importance, but the function of the hand is essential. The hand may look cosmetically good after surgery but may lose its function. On the other hand, if pain is an outstanding symptom, then surgery should be a consideration.

Artificial replacement of the small joints of the hands has been done through brilliant engineering concepts. Ideally the operation should provide normal range of motion, a balance of the tendons about the joint against future subluxations, and durability. With the use of silicone and small joint replacements, some of these goals have been achieved. The primary problem of joint replacement in the hand is the maintenance of the bone that is already there, as some of the bone may continue to be destroyed by stresses and the illness.

A rheumatoid hand may be severely deformed, ugly in appearance, but can still be useful to the owner. Surgery may remove the remaining function the patient has; the hand may look cosmetically better, but the function is worse.

Prior to undertaking hand surgery, a second opinion is necessary. A thorough evaluation of the underlying disease must be researched: how much rheumatoid arthritis and how long. Has every medical means been exhausted? The surgeon doing corrective hand surgery must be experienced in this operation.

Total Hip Replacement or Total Joint Arthroplasty (Due to Arthritis)

John Charniley, an Englishman, carried out the first total hip arthroplasty at the Mayo Clinic in March of 1969.

The patient must realize that total replacement of the hip joint has a certain amount of finality to it because a considerable amount of bone and joint is removed in order to insert the artificial joint. If failure occurs, re-operation is a very difficult and serious proposition.

The recovery period is short, is relatively painless, and early results are almost uniformly good. We can anticipate 95 percent of patients will have good results in the early years, but as time goes on, mechanical and biological failure of these implants occurs, which may range from 25 percent at five years to 50 percent at the end of ten years.

The Indications for Total Hip Replacement

Pain is the outstanding indication. Patients generally have a limp, use a cane or crutches, and are limited in the distance they can walk. They have difficulty climbing stairs, rising from a chair, or driving a car, and are unable to put on shoes and socks. The disability takes into account the way in which pain and restriction of function affect the patient.

X-ray examination may show a very deteriorated hip, yet the patient may have minimal symptoms. The disability that the patient exhibits should determine whether or not hip replacement should be performed, not the X ray.

Cautions Prior to Doing Hip Replacement

As in all general surgical procedures, the patient must be in optimal health, not suffering from serious pulmonary or cardiac illness. A thorough medical evaluation is performed. Any infections anywhere in the body, whether dental or genitourinary, must be corrected. Many surgeons request the presence of an internist for medical clearance prior to surgery.

Pre-Operative Evaluation

In addition to giving the patient a thorough medical examination, the physician should look for infection in the joint itself. It is desirable, and in some cases mandatory, that a joint aspiration be performed before surgery, with a culture of fluid from the joint to determine if there are any infections.

Patients who only have X-ray findings and stiffness and minimal pain should not be operated on. If a surgeon advises an operation, a second opinion is mandatory.

Patients must understand that they can never engage in running or jumping sports, and will be limited in extensive stair climbing, but will be able to walk, do light housework and bench work. Patients do very well with the new hip: they can swim, bike-ride, and bowl without pain. Hip surgery can prevent confinement to a wheelchair. Recently, young children suffering from rheumatoid arthritis have had total replacement with success.

12: Thyroid Surgery

THYROID GLAND

OUTSIDE PARIS, in a small secluded village, stood the Château St. Aetinne, surrounded by elegant carriages and spacious lawns. The tall windows are barred and it is snowing. The year is 1830.

In some of the rooms, the windows are flung open as elegant ladies parade naked, screaming, prancing back and forth wringing their hands in despair, complaining of the heat as the snowflakes enter. Their eyes are popping. They are thin, emaciated like the witches from *Macbeth*. In other rooms women are lying in bed with their wrists and feet tied down, covered by cold blankets as they lie in delirium, muttering nonsense and vulgarities.

In the parlor women are talking in loud tones, their thoughts racing ahead of them, stumbling on words, anxious, nervous, worrying that there are people who are about to kill them, eating voraciously from plates piled with pheasant, beef, fried potatoes, and pudding.

This description is not from the pages of the Marquis de Sade, but from notes of Dr. Basedow, who established a rest home for affluent Victorian ladies suffering from overactive thyroids, for whom no treatment was available except relaxation, rest, and trials of seaweed and burnt sponge. When they survived, some of the women became normal (euthyroid), others developed an underactive thyroid (hypothyroidism, myxedema), and were described as follows:

"In the other part of the house, women are lying around listless, covered with wool blankets, with puffy face, puffy eyes, thin hair on their eyelids, pale, anemic, semi-comatous, and some frankly insane."

This historical description of overactive thyroid disease enables us today to perceive the natural course of this illness: after running a long, stormy course, the thyroid can return to normal with no treatment; others burn their thyroid out and then it becomes underactive; other times the patient dies.

The Anatomy and Physiology of the Thyroid Gland

The thyroid gland was first described by Vesalius in the sixteenth century. The name comes from the Greek word *thureos* or *shield*. Described as like a butterfly in shape, this very important gland is located in the neck, straddling the windpipe, surrounded by nerves that help control the motion of the voice box. Enmeshed in its center are other structures called the parathyroid glands, which govern the metabolism of calcium in the body.

The thyroid gland earned its reputation by secreting hormones called *thyroxine* and *triiodothyronine,* which govern the metabolism of the body. Its secretions depend on the continuous stimulation from the master gland (pituitary) by the thyroid-stimulating hormone. When the thyroid gland manufactures enough hormones, it blocks the secretion of the thyroid-stimulating hormone, which then decreases further hormone release from the thyroid. The entire system is governed by a still higher control, called the *hypothalamus,* in the brain.

The thyroid relies on iodine to manufacture the hormones thyroxine and triiodothyronine. In adults the thyroid weighs between 15 and 20 grams, sometimes weighing up to 50 grams. Lack of iodine going to the gland causes enlargement of the gland, or *goiter.* The disease of the thyroid will be discussed from a medical and a surgical point of view in regard to its overactivity, called *hyperthyroidism;* the tumefaction of the gland, called *goiter;* and growths of the thyroid that are benign and cancerous.

HYPERTHYROIDISM OR OVERACTIVE THYROID

Summary of Symptoms of Overactive Thyroid

An overactive thyroid can cause a voracious appetite with accompanying weight loss, intolerance to heat, shaking, tremors, increased thirst, diarrhea, and fast heartbeat—sometimes so fast that the heart may go into failure. If untreated it may progress to a thyroid storm, as evidenced by temperatures of 105, delirium, heart failure, and death.

Laboratory Diagnosis of Thyroid Disease

Not too long ago the diagnosis of overactive thyroid (hyperthyroidism) or underactive thyroid (hypothyroidism) was determined by a test called the BMR (basal metabolism rate). Today the actual level of thyroid hormones can be measured with blood tests, including the hormone from the pituitary, called the thyroid-stimulating hormone.

Other tests consist of the radioactive iodine uptake and radioisotope scanning. This combined test gives information on the functioning, size, and position of the gland. All medications containing iodine products must be discontinued. An isotope is injected and the scan begins in a few minutes with a Geiger counter over the gland to measure the activity in the uptake. This test enables us to determine if the gland is overactive, underactive, or whether it contains abnormal growths. This is the same type of procedure that is used to perform bone scans and liver scans. This test is followed by no discomfort or pain and has no aftereffects.

The Treatment of Hyperthyroidism

There are medical treatment, radiation therapy, and surgery.

THE MEDICAL TREATMENT

The medical man feels hyperthyroidism is his domain and uses appropriate drugs, called antithyroid drugs, to treat this condition.

Iodine is the oldest remedy for disorders of the thyroid gland. During the nineteenth and early twentieth centuries, iodine was used for overactive thyroid and goiters. The response to administering iodine in overactive thyroids is dramatic and impressive within the first twenty-four hours. The release of the hormone from the thyroid gland into the circulation is rapidly interrupted, the maximum effect being achieved in two weeks. Unfortunately, iodine therapy usually does not completely control the manifestations of overactive thyroid, and beneficial effects seem to wear off after a little time. For this reason iodine as the sole agent was abandoned and is only used before surgery in the treatment of this disorder.

Medications to prevent the actual formation of thyroid hormones was introduced in 1941. These medications, called *thiourea,* are used to this day.

The medical treatment is effective in the majority of patients. Experience has taught us that the optimal time for treatment is a year. Unfortunately, 40 percent of the time the thyroid again becomes overactive after the treatment is discontinued and treatment must be reinstated.

Sometimes treatment is administered indefinitely. Most patients tolerate the medication well and side effects are few, but there is the constant expense associated with taking the medications. Because of the prolonged treatment and inconvenience to the patient, radiation treatment was devised.

If the thyroid is very large and there is danger of compression, surgery is necessary. In most cases only a small portion of the gland is enlarged, and today most endocrinologists oppose surgery. If surgery is advocated, a second opinion is needed.

Surgical removal of an overactive thyroid raises the possibility of serious complications and death, although these are rare. Destruction of the nerve surrounding the thyroid causes paralysis of the voice box, and the danger of removing the parathyroid glands, which are essential to life for calcium metabolism. Finally, patients will need permanent thyroid replacement. Surgery is costly and requires hospitalization.

Today there is general agreement among physicians that the best treatment for hyperthyroidism is not surgery but either medication or radiation. Radiation is gaining popularity in women past childbearing age.

Surgery is performed on a woman of childbearing age when medical management fails or the patient just doesn't take her medications.

RADIATION TREATMENT OF HYPERTHYROIDISM
RADIOACTIVE IODINE (RAI)

The RAI treatment is currently the most popular and most frequently used method of therapy. The dosage is administered orally in a half-glass of water. The effective dose varies in individual patients and depends on the size of the gland.

After treatment with this method there is progressive recovery and few untoward effects. Treatment failures are rare and there is a permanent cure, which may appear after a variable interval of a few days to a few weeks, the symptoms of an overactive thyroid abating entirely in two or three months. Further treatment sometimes is necessary at the end of three months.

The advantages of this treatment are that it is easy to administer, is less costly than surgery, can be given on an outpatient basis, and is almost 100 percent curative when given in the correct dosage. It is, however, associated with a high percentage of patients whose thyroids become underactive, hypothyroid. This method of thyroid ablation remains the popular mode but should not be used during pregnancy. Some thyroidologists claim that birth defects and cancer may result from this form of treatment. However, extensive studies have failed to show the validity of either of these complications. The major disadvantage is that 20 percent of patients may have to be treated subsequently with thyroid hormones.

At the present time many endocrinologists begin treatment of an overactive thyroid with medication. If the patient is elderly and has congestive heart failure or a rapid heart rate, the medical man fully agrees that radioactive iodine is the best treatment. If repeated attempts by medical treatment fail, then radioactive iodine is also indicated.

Surgical Treatment of Overactive Thyroid: The Surgeon's View

Surgery provides definitive treatment of this illness. Prolonged medical care is avoided and there is no risk of radiation. In expert hands this operation rarely has complications and the mortality rate is exceedingly low. If there is a large gland pressing on the trachea (windpipe), causing breathing difficulties, surgery must be performed. Medical treatment or radiation may control the symptoms of an overactive thyroid, but the disfiguring appearance of an enlarged thyroid remains.

Patients are reminded each morning as they look in the mirror of the unattractiveness of their necks. They are constantly rearranging their wardrobe to hide the deformity. Necklaces only highlight the swelling. Many female patients find this unacceptable and would rather have a tiny scar than a protruding mass in the neck.

GOITER

Iodine is needed to manufacture thyroid hormones. A deficiency of iodine leads to enlargement of the thyroid gland, called goiter.

Prevalence of Goiter

Goiter was once widely prevalent in countries like Switzerland, Austria, southern Germany, and northern Spain and was first described by the Swiss-German physician, Paracelsus, in the sixteenth century in Salzburg, Austria. Paracelsus, who was a brilliant physician and pharmacologist, identified mental retardation and cretinism due to an enlarged goiter.

Goiter is a rare disease in our society. In areas where severe iodine deficiency is present, virtually everyone is goiterous regardless of age or sex. The gland seems suddenly to enlarge in early childhood and puberty. Females are generally affected more than males, as in all thyroid conditions. In certain endemic areas, such as New Guinea, thyroid enlargement may actually follow breast enlargement.

There may be genetic influences on goiter formation in small groups of patients. These genetic abnormalities result in the inability of the thyroid gland to trap the badly needed iodine necessary to manufacture the hormones, or the inability to convert the iodine into a form that can be used. There are goitrogenic substances that cause goiter, as cabbage, turnips, brussels sprouts, and soybean milk in infants. Chemical substances may also cause goiters; for example, salts and minerals like lithium and cobalt have been found to cause goiters. In the United States goiters are rare, as most table salt has added iodine.

Symptoms of Goiter

Goiters, as a rule, are not overactive or underactive in function. They may achieve a large size and cause pressure symptoms such as coughing, wheezing, and swallowing difficulties. Patients may notice a swelling in their necks, or it is discovered by the physician.

Usually goiters cause no symptoms and are only of aesthetic importance. Occasionally goiters are found extending into the chest. These are most troublesome, as they can cause respiratory problems by their compression on the windpipe.

Treatment of Goiter

It was known for centuries that iodine-containing substances were helpful in treating swellings of the neck, such as seaweed and burnt sponge, mentioned previously. In 1817 Bernard Courtois, a French manufacturer of saltpeter, discovered iodine. Tincture of iodine was first used for the treatment of goiter in 1870.

Some endocrinologists favor the thyroid hormone to be given to all goiter sufferers to suppress the thyroid-stimulating hormone in order to prevent further growth of the goiter or the rare complication of hemorrhage into the gland. A thyroid goiter is removed for the following reasons: 1) When there are symptoms of compression: respiratory or swallowing difficulties; and 2) for cosmetic reasons.

Studies have failed to provide convincing evidence of cancer formation in a goiter.

If the two criteria above are not met when surgery is advised, a second opinion is needed.

THE THYROID NODULE

The management of a solitary growth or nodule of the thyroid remains a highly controversial issue among surgeons and medical men because of the fear that these nodules are cancerous. The thyroid nodule, in contrast to the goiter, is a growth of thyroid tissue in the form of a nodule. The incidence of a thyroid cancer in a single nodule is four times the probability of that in a goiter.

The Pathophysiology of Thyroid Nodules

Thyroid nodules, as a rule, are nonfunctional: not over- or underactive. We have discussed toxic thyroid nodules, or hyperthyroidism. As a general rule, when these nodules are not functioning, there is a greater tendency for them to be cancerous.

Factors That Predispose Thyroid Cancer in the Nodule

If a nodule occurs in a male, it is more likely to be malignant than a nodule occurring in a female. Half of the thyroid nodules appearing in children are malignant (80 percent of children with carcinoma of the thyroid are found to have had previous neck radiation). Any previous radiation to the head and neck increases the likelihood of cancer in that nodule.

The Physical Examination

A nodule harboring a cancer has certain suspicious characteristics. History of recent thyroid growth and difficulty swallowing or breathing should make the physician suspicious. If the nodule is stony hard, not freely movable, and lymph glands are palpable, then cancer should be suspected.

Laboratory Examination

Blood tests are performed to determine if this nodule is hyperactive, overactive, or nonfunctioning. A radioactive scan of the thyroid is employed to see if the nodule is "cold" or "hot" or normal. A cold nodule means it has no activity or function and raises the suspicion of cancer. A hot nodule means an overactive gland.

Most thyroid cancers are found to have cold nodules. A thyroid scan cannot be used to differentiate between a benign and a malignant nodule and the results of one should not be a criterion for surgery.

Ultrasound

Ultrasound is also used in trying to differentiate between a solid nodule and a cyst. Cysts have been reported to occur in 20 percent of nodules. There is less incidence of cancer in a cystic lesion than in a solid nodule. Despite the useful information that might be obtained to differentiate the different types of nodules, ultrasound should also not be used to make the final decision on whether the nodule should be removed.

Needle Biopsy of the Thyroid Gland

This is a simple procedure performed in the physician's office, sometimes not even requiring local anesthesia. It involves simply taking a syringe with a needle at its end and aspirating substance from this nodule. The tissue is then studied. Negative biopsy does not rule out cancer: the needle can sample a normal tissue adjacent to the cancer. Ninety percent of needle biopsies in one series diagnosed cancer confirmed at surgery.

Treatment of the Solitary Nodule: The Surgical Point of View

A suspicious nodule should be removed rather than have the patient spend years in medical treatment. The patient lives in constant fear that cancer may be present. Prolonged cost of medication and medical treatment is necessary without surgery. In expert hands, thyroid surgery has few risks and complications.

All thyroid nodules found in patients who give a history of radiation during infancy should be removed surgically, as the chance of a cancer being present is strong. Thyroid nodules that have the characteristics of cancer, namely, those which are stony hard and not movable and have already spread to adjacent lymph nodes, should also be removed.

Medical Point of View

All thyroid nodules should be investigated, but not all need to be removed surgically. An example of a recent patient comes to mind.

A twenty-four-year-old female with a thyroid nodule which was freely movable was seen in our office. All the tests indicated that it was not active. A needle aspiration was performed; the biopsy was negative. The surgeon had decided to operate on the nodule and the patient was scheduled for surgery in the coming three weeks. During this time the thyroid nodule slowly, progressively decreased in size and disappeared after the aspiration, and the surgery was canceled.

If the thyroid nodule is nonfunctioning or cold, and aspiration does not reveal evidence of malignancy, thyroid hormone suppression should be attempted for three months. Again, if the thyroid nodule disappears, treatment is continued. If after a period of three months the nodule does not decrease in size, then surgery should be performed.

THYROID CARCINOMA

We have just discussed a nodule in the thyroid which may or may not be cancerous. The next discussion will center on definitive thyroid cancers. This is another highly complicated subject. For example, certain minimal thyroid cancers, called *papillary thyroid carcinomas,* have a negligible risk, while others, like anaplastic carcinoma of the thyroid, are among the worst malignancies possible.

The following is a useful classification of the types of thyroid cancer. The classification is made according to their behavior.

1. Papillary thyroid cancers occur in all age groups. It is three times more common in females than in males and represents the great majority of thyroid cancers seen in adults and children. It is a slow-growing tumor of low-grade malignancy.

2. Follicular cancer spreads through the blood and occurs in old age groups. It accounts for about 30 percent of cancers in females and is more common in women than in men. These tumors metastasize through the bloodstream rather than the lymph nodes as in papillary cancers. They occur between the ages of thirty and sixty.

3. Undifferentiated thyroid cancers (anaplastic carcinoma) occur predominantly in older patients and kill by a local spread. There is only a 1 percent survival after ten years. Death generally results from local spread before distant metastases occur.

The effects and outcome of cancers, particularly papillary and follicular cancers, depend on the age of the patient, the extent of the tumor, the presence of distant spread, whether they invade the blood, and the sex of the patient.

If all thyroid glands were studied at autopsy, ten to thirty million persons would have evidence of minimal papillary thyroid cancer. Deaths from tumors of the thyroid are uncommon compared with other cancers as, for example, cancer of the colon and bowel.

Predisposition to Developing Thyroid Cancers

External radiation, mentioned earlier, is associated with increased incidence of thyroid cancers. When overactive thyroid, or thyrotoxicosis, is treated with therapeutic radiation, there is no increase of cancer because the thyroid cells are completely destroyed. However, low doses of irradiation can induce cancer. That is why it is so important to have a correct dosage range in treating thyrotoxicosis with radiation. It has been estimated that the interval between radiation to the thyroid gland and the appearance of cancer may be from twenty-five to thirty-five years and as short as three and a half years.

Thyroid cancer is three times more common in females than in males, occurring in a peak incidence in the sixth decade, from infancy to old age.

Treatment of Thyroid Cancer

The treatment of thyroid cancer is subtotal thyroid removal. However, if there is extension into the neck, more radical surgery is required.

Surgery of Papillary Carcinoma

Controversy rages on whether a complete removal of the thyroid, called a total thyroidectomy, be performed, or only the thyroid lobe removed on one side. Radical total thyroidectomy means the removal of the main muscle of the neck, sacrificing the nerve that goes to the shoulders, and removal of the jugular vein, plus complete removal of the thyroid gland. Some of the conspicuous results of this surgery are deformity of the neck, a drooping of the shoulder, troublesome arthritis, a significant mortality rate, plus a very disfiguring scar left on the neck. The incidence of removal of the parathyroid gland, along with the thyroid, ranges from 15 to 20 percent, and in competent hands may be 10 percent. The complications of removal of the parathyroid gland are severe cramps in the legs, convulsions, tetany, and early cataracts.

The major argument against removing the entire thyroid is the extensive surgery required, the risk of nerve paralysis, and the results of an underactive parathyroid gland. There is no evidence that extensive operation on the neck to remove the total thyroid improved survival rates or reduced recurrences. There is a 40 to 50 percent complication rate when thyroids are removed completely; there is only a 13 percent complication rate when part of the thyroid is removed. In addition, it has been found that if there is distant spread of the tumor, then radiation therapy with I31 should be given. Dosages of radioactive iodine should be given after surgery in patients with papillary carcinoma. In case the patient is not operable, thyroid hormones should be given to prolong the actual survival time to eleven years.

Inoperable cancer of the thyroid may occur if the cancer is too far spread or if the patient is in too poor medical condition to have surgery.

Follicular Carcinoma

This is a much more serious tumor and must be treated aggressively, as spread through the blood occurs frequently. Thyroidectomy is necessary, followed by radioactive iodine therapy and lifelong thyroid hormone replacement.

Anaplastic Cancer of the Thyroid

Very often these cancers are so malignant that they compress the airway tract, the trachea, making breathing impossible. Radical surgery performed for follicular carcinoma should not be done, but a simple procedure should be employed with external radiation to the neck.

Other cancers of the thyroid which have not been discussed, like medullary carcinoma of the thyroid, are very rare.

13: *Stomach Surgery: Ulcer, Cancer of the Stomach, Diaphragmatic Hernia (Hiatal Hernia)*

ULCER DISEASE

ON A MORNING in March 1822 a French-Canadian by the name of Alexis St. Martin was wounded at close range by a shotgun blast that tore open his lower chest and abdomen, lacerating the stomach badly. The wound was filled with blood, bone splinters, lead shot, bits of clothing, and contents of the stomach. This accident occurred in Fort Michilimackinac in northern Michigan. An obscure army surgeon by the name of William Beaumont, who had learned medicine through an apprenticeship, was called to treat the dying man. It appeared that the wound was fatal, but Beaumont cleaned it, dressed it, made his patient comfortable, and, miraculously, after a lengthy convalescence the patient survived but was left with a permanent opening giving direct view to his stomach—a fistula.

Beaumont brought his patient nearly two thousand miles to the Plattsburgh Barracks, New York, where he was able to study the digestion and movement of the stomach. He observed the stomach secrete juices and found the gastric juice contained hydrochloric acid. Beaumont was the true leader and pioneer of experimental physiology in our country. This Connecticut physician received only limited recognition in America, while European scientists held his work as a major accomplishment. His observations led to the understanding of how in some patients the excess free acid in the stomach breaks the protective barrier, causing some to have a chronic irritation called gastritis, while others experience an actual destruction of the lining.

Definition and Anatomy

The stomach has the form of a Spanish skin wine flask. Ulcers appearing in the body of the flask are called gastric ulcers; those at the exit of the flask, pyloric ulcers; and those at the first portion of the small intestine, duodenal ulcers.

Incidence of the Disease

In the United States, it is estimated about three million people are affected by peptic ulcers each year; 600,000 of them have gastric ulcers and 2.4 million have duodenal ulcers. Gastric ulcers seem to occur in older people more often than duodenal ulcers, and there has been a significant decrease in the incidence of both. The precise process that results in gastric and duodenal ulcerations is still not fully understood.

The Symptoms of Duodenal Ulcers

The classical symptom of duodenal ulcers is pain in the upper portion of the stomach, occurring two to three hours or more after meals, in the late afternoon, or at night, and relieved by food or antacids. Clusters of episodes occurring, lasting for days or weeks, are interspersed with pain-free intervals of weeks or months.

Gastric Ulcers

Gastric ulcers are characterized by chronic and periodic pain in the upper portion of the abdomen, but the symptom pattern is less predictable than for duodenal lesions. Pain before or after meals may or may not be relieved by antacids but may be associated with nausea or vomiting. Weight loss is commonly encountered.

Diagnosis of peptic ulcers characteristically rests on a GI series with the visualization of the stomach and duodenum. More precise diagnoses are accomplished through endoscopy, in which a well-constructed flexible instrument is passed into the stomach.

Endoscopic Examination of the Upper Gastrointestinal Tract

A flexible tube is guided through the patient's mouth into the stomach after sedation has been administered; the patient does not eat or drink for several hours before the test. A topical anesthetic is applied to the patient's throat.

The endoscope is a system of optic fibers that transmit light into the instrument and into the area under view. The endoscope has openings that allow biopsies to be performed if necessary and fluid to be aspirated. Pictures of the interior can be taken. This examination can be performed in fifteen minutes, but sometimes may last as long as an hour, either in the hospital room, in the emergency room, or in the doctor's office. The risk of this procedure is the slight possibility of perforation of the esophagus.

The Indications for Endoscopic Examination

If X-ray proof of the diagnosis of ulcer is lacking, and if after a prescribed form of treatment there is no improvement, endoscopic examination is indicated. A GI series can miss 20 percent of duodenal ulcers. If X ray demonstrates a gastric ulcer, the radiological differentiation between a benign ulcer and a cancer of the stomach may be impossible. Endoscopy is generally performed for direct visualization and biopsy. Endoscopic examination may alone miss a cancer of the stomach unless accompanied with a brushing of the ulcer to obtain cells and biopsy.

Another indication for performing endoscopy is when pain becomes refractory to medical management and surgery is contemplated.

If a GI series demonstrates a duodenal ulcer, there is no need to perform endoscopy, which is a costly procedure reserved for specific indications and which should not be abused for indiscriminate routine scoping.

Complications of Ulcer Disease

1. Perforation, in which a hole is made through the stomach by the acid and empties its contents into the abdomen.
2. Progressive scar formation from a recurrent ulcer, causing obstruction of the outlet of the stomach.
3. Hemorrhage.
4. The failure of the ulcer to heal.

Endoscopy should not be performed if a perforation of the stomach is suspected, but if there is vomiting of blood, endoscopy can determine more accurately than a GI series the site in 80 to 90 percent of patients.

Treatment of Peptic Ulcers

Most patients improve with the standard known treatment of antacids, which attempt to neutralize excessive acids. Pliny the

Elder, in ancient times, prescribed milk for the treatment of gastric distress. Milk has survived as the choice of treatment for thousands of years, until recently; it has been discovered that milk is not the ideal treatment as it causes rebound of acid formation. A new drug called cimetidine (Tagamet) has made an enormous impact on ulcer disease. By a dramatic reduction in production of acid, it has diminished significantly the complications of ulcers, and "intractable ulcers" are becoming less common.

Intense nervousness, anxiety, cigarette smoking, aspirin and aspirin compounds, and alcohol in excess can prevent healing of an ulcer. Unfortunately, the doctor may fail to advise the patient to eliminate aspirin and wonder why the ulcer becomes intractable.

In spite of the excellent treatment, peptic disease still accounts for seventy-five hundred deaths per year and forty thousand disabled individuals with an estimated economic loss as high as $3.2 billion each year. Ulcers have a reputation as something to be taken lightly or to joke about, especially in the old-time movies, when it was a favorite form of derision.

Surgical Indications for the Treatment of Ulcer Disease

If there is perforation, severe obstruction, or uncontrolled hemorrhage, surgery must be performed promptly. If a patient has intractable, disabling pain, surgery can be considered.

The Choice of Operation of Removal of the Stomach

Ever since the first recorded operation in 1635 by a surgeon called Mathis from Prague, in which he tried to remove a knife from the stomach of a peasant, numerous operations have been devised. The most widely performed operation today is called a vagotomy and pyloroplasty. The vagus nerve, which mediates acid production of the stomach, is cut and the outlet of the stomach is widened to allow rapid emptying. This is associated with few side effects, but there is a 10 percent chance of recurrence of the ulcer.

There are several variations of the operation, as when the vagus nerve is cut and the lower third of the stomach is removed; or the newer operation, gaining in popularity, in which the vagus nerve is removed from the upper part of the stomach where acid is made and the nerves in the lower part of the stomach and intestines are left intact. This latter operation is becoming popular, as it avoids the troublesome aftereffect of chronic diarrhea, and reduces recurrence rates of ulcer to less than 5 percent.

The Medical Opinion

After exhaustive medical treatment for duodenal ulcer disease, consisting of cessation of smoking, antacids, and a new medication, cimetidine, then stomach surgery can be considered. If there is perforation of the stomach or obstruction, surgery remains the choice of treatment. Most bleeding from the gastrointestinal tract can be controlled by conservative treatment. When the bleeding becomes so profuse that it cannot be controlled, then surgery is mandatory to save the life of the patient. Some gastroenterologists favor surgery if bleeding fails to cease after 6 to 8 units of blood have been given. Death from ulcer occurs from massive hemorrhage and perforation of the stomach.

Gastric Ulcer

In many patients an X ray of the stomach cannot reveal whether the gastric ulcer is benign or cancerous, and gastroscopic examination must be performed. A gastric ulcer that does not heal after twelve weeks requires surgery because of the possibility of malignancy.

CANCER OF THE STOMACH

The good news concerning cancer of the stomach is that it is on the decline in industrial countries, for reasons which are obscure. Recently it has been reported to be on the decline in France, while in countries like Japan, Iceland, and Finland it seems to be on the increase. Some investigators feel that the Japanese consume large quantities of smoked fish and this possibly has a causal relationship to the disease. Diets high in starch and low in fresh fruits and vegetables have been thought to bring on stomach cancers. This disease occurs in men more often than women, in the ratio of 2:1, the peak incidence occurring in the fifty to fifty-nine age group. Jack Benny was a recent victim of stomach cancer.

Predisposition to Cancer of the Stomach

In past years stomach ulcers were believed to be forerunners of stomach cancer, but this has been disproven. One disease closely associated with cancer is pernicious anemia. This disease is a blood disorder characterized by the inability to absorb vitamin B_{12}; its victims' stomachs have no acid and do not secrete a protein called the intrinsic factor, necessary for B_{12} absorption. Vitamin B_{12} injections control this disease.

Symptoms of Cancer of the Stomach

Symptoms are nonspecific, vague, sometimes resembling ulcer pain in character, and include burning not relieved by antacids. There is loss of appetite and weakness accompanying the stomach symptoms. As a rule there may be no symptoms for a long period of time except for general discomfort or vague feelings in the chest and stomach. The outstanding symptom may result from blood loss or anemia, consistent with weakness and fatigue and not corrected by over-the-counter "tired blood" medications.

Diagnosis for Cancer of the Stomach

The GI series, already mentioned, may show a characteristic finding of the gastric cancer. The endoscope, mentioned earlier, with the study of cells and biopsy remains the most accurate diagnostic procedure.

The most common malignancy of the stomach begins in the inside lining, called *adenocarcinoma.*

Treatment of this illness is radical surgery and chemotherapy. Dr. Theodore Bilroth from Vienna devised the procedure in 1890, called the Bilroth II operation, which removed a good portion of the stomach. Larger cancers necessitate removal of the entire organ.

The stressful aftereffect of the operation is called the dumping syndrome: the stomach empties rapidly, causing nausea, sweating, faintness, and weakness, following any meal. In 90 percent of patients this dumping syndrome subsides within six months.

The bad news is that most patients suffering from cancer of the stomach die in two years. More recently, with earlier diagnosis using the gastroscope and with chemotherapy, survival is prolonged.

HIATAL HERNIAS (SLIDING HERNIAS)

Heartburn is a nasty symptom, especially the kind that occurs only when bending down or in the middle of the night and feels like a heart attack—sometimes it is a heart attack. This burning, searing sensation that feels like someone placed a hot poker down into the gut after a night of drinking or spicy foods has many causes, such as ulcer disease, inflammation of the stomach, gastritis, and a hiatal hernia.

A hiatal hernia simply means the stomach is sliding into the chest (whereas the stomach is separated from the chest by the diaphragm, it sometimes parades upward into the chest). If, as it ascends, it also causes acid to regurgitate, heartburn follows.

Acids flow up from the stomach into the esophagus because the valve mechanism at the end of the stomach does not work properly.

Diaphragmatic hernia, or a hiatal hernia, is a common finding on a GI series. These hiatal hernias are considered to be of two types: 1) sliding (axial), which make up 90 percent of the hernias, in which the stomach moves straight upward, and 2) para-esophageal, in which the stomach rotates alongside the esophagus.

Once the diagnosis of a diaphragmatic hernia is made, no treatment is generally required. However, if there is evidence of regurgitation—namely, acid flowing upward, with the symptoms of heartburn, indigestion, and chest pain—then it can be a symptomatic diaphragmatic hernia, which requires treatment.

The Diagnosis of Diaphragmatic Hernia That Causes Reflux

It must first be shown that the esophagus suffers from reflux of the gastric juice. Several tests are performed: 1) a reflux PH probe test, which measures the actual acidity that flows to the esophagus; 2) the Bernstein test, in which a small amount of hydrochloric acid is placed down into the esophagus and the patient is asked if he feels the heartburn. This test then tells us that the reflux of acid causes the symptom in the first place and the esophagus is sensitive to the acid; 3) a motility study is done by measuring the various pressures and motion of the esophagus, especially the lower esophagus, to see if the lower valve is functioning properly.

The Medical Treatment of Diaphragmatic Hernia

The treatment consists of neutralization of the acid by ingestion of liquid antacids; at night the head of the bed needs to be elevated to prevent the regurgitation of acid. Food should not be eaten for three to four hours before bedtime. Recently,

Tagamet has been used with some success. Spicy foods may bring on the pain as well as smoking and alcohol.

The Surgical Treatment of Diaphragmatic Hernia

The indication for operations on diaphragmatic hernias is severe, unrelenting pain. Before an operation is performed, it must be shown, with the tests described, that the esophagus suffers from reflux of gastric juice.

If in spite of the elimination of offending agents, such as coffee, alcohol, and spicy substances, and the use of antacid treatment, the burning becomes severe and there is danger of stricture or hemorrhage, then surgery should be performed.

Para-esophageal hernias may bleed. The bleeding is usually slow but does not stop with medical treatment, and surgery is indicated.

14: *Cancer of the Colon, Diverticulosis, and Diverticulitis*

CANCER OF THE COLON

HE WAS A FIFTY-EIGHT-YEAR-OLD FAMILY MAN, who one morning after a bowel movement saw some blood in the toilet bowl. Fearful to tell anyone, he went to work at the plant and put the whole matter out of his mind. Each morning for weeks he searched for the blood and, when he saw none, was relieved. Finally months later he told his wife how weak he felt. The cancer was discovered, spread to other parts of his body, and he was doomed. Later he confessed to the doctor he had seen the blood many times the year before.

Another patient, sixty years old, who was health conscious, watched his diet carefully, had given up smoking five years before, and exercised regularly, found some blood in his stool one morning. That same day he went to see his physician, who examined him, discovered hemorrhoids, and prescribed some ointment. The bleeding ceased and then restarted, but the patient felt assured they were bleeding hemorrhoids. He died two years later of cancer of the rectum that had spread to all parts of his body. The physician had failed to do more tests and the cancer was discovered too late.

A shy, reserved fifty-year-old man, successful in business, went for his yearly company physical, having every test performed, including an exercise stress test, chest X ray, blood tests, and pulmonary function test—everything except a rectal examination.

"I can't stand that exam," he told his doctor, and refused it each time. He, too, harbored a slow-growing cancer of the rectum, easily within reach of the examining finger, and died several years later.

Still another patient with no symptoms at all was found to have a polyp of the intestine on a routine physical examination which included a rectal examination and a sigmoidoscopy. The doctor advised removal of the polyp but the patient refused and went to see no other physician. Eight years later the patient died of spread of cancer of the bowel.

More recently, a patient saw one of the authors because of shortness of breath when climbing the stairs. She was a nurse, who, when questioned, denied any symptoms of bowel habit changes, weight loss, nausea, or vomiting, admitting only to weakness and shortness of breath. The physical examination was entirely normal, including the rectal examination and sigmoidoscopy, but she was found to have a very low blood count: she was anemic. Further diagnostic tests revealed that she had cancer on the right side of her large intestine. She was operated on and her outlook is good.

These brief anecdotes are all true stories from our case book, and they summarize the problem of this cancer in the United States, a disease that kills twenty-five thousand men and twenty-seven thousand women yearly. This is the most prevalent cancer in the United States, with an estimated 112,000 new cases reported in 1979. It is the second most common cause of death from cancer (lung cancer heads the list). Many of these 112,000 patients could be saved with early diagnosis and treatment. There is little controversy about what is expected of the physician and of the patient for the correct steps in detecting this illness. The patient who has a rectal bleed should insist upon proper examination.

The patient who has an annual physical should have a rectal examination with stool test for blood. It is the patient's responsibility to report abnormal bleeding to his or her physician and to discuss fears and realize that in 1980 cancer is a controllable disease and, many times, curable. Twenty-five percent of all cancers of the rectum begin in the portion of the rectum that can be palpated by a doctor's examining finger. Another 50 percent can be seen through the sigmoidoscope, a long lighted tube that is inserted into the anus.

Risk Factors and Possible Causes

There are some patients who are more susceptible to developing cancer of the large intestine and rectum than others. Blood relatives of patients with this cancer have a higher risk than those with families in which the disease has not occurred. Women who have had breast cancer or cancer of the uterus, or cervix, also have a higher than normal risk. Polyps of the large intestine mean an increased incidence of cancer.

What Are Polyps?

A polyp is a raised growth rising from the inner lining of the large intestine that may already contain cancer cells if they are larger than 1 cm. If these polyps are greater than 2 cm, the risk of cancer may be 40 percent.

Polyps run in families: some members develop cancer at an average age of thirty-nine, and some even develop in children under the age of sixteen. Other family members of any individual who is found with this diagnosis are carefully examined.

Some cancer specialists propose complete removal of the bowel, called a colectomy; others advocate six-month careful examinations with removal only of the polyps.

Patients who get a chronic inflammation of the small intestine extending into the large intestine, referred to as Crohn's disease or terminal ileitis, are twenty times more likely to develop cancer of the colon. People with ulcerative colitis, an inflammatory disease of the large intestine, causing bloody diarrhea, have a 3 to 5 percent risk of developing cancer of the colon ten years after the initial diagnosis is made.

Cancer of the terminal portion of the digestive tract or large bowel is another price to pay for living in Western culture, except in Finland. Japan, parts of Asia, Africa, and most of South America, with the exception of Uruguay and Argentina, have a low incidence of cancer of the large bowel. As the Japanese have migrated to the United States, they develop more large bowel cancer as compared with their fellow countrymen in Japan. American blacks develop more cancer than African blacks.

Epidemiological studies have strongly suggested that the dietary habits of our culture and the other cultures play a significant role in this observed disparity. Foods low in animal fat and refined carbohydrates, and high in bulk, vegetables, and fruits seem to protect the colon from cancer (foods associated with frequent defecation or, as the gastroenterologists say, rapid transit time). Dietary fats seem to alter the concentrations of substances such as bile acid and cholesterol, in the bowel.

As yet no specific cancer-producing product in our food substances has been identified that causes the cancer. It remains to be seen if changing our dietary habits to include bulk while eliminating meat and increasing vegetables and fruits will decrease our incidence of bowel cancer.

Symptoms and Detection of Cancer of the Large Intestine and Rectum

In our initial case histories we have already mentioned the symptom of rectal bleeding, which may be the only symptom. Sometimes it may be a dramatic hemorrhage with the patient first seen in the emergency room. There may be no symptoms until the disease has spread to other organs or the patient complains of change of bowel habits, suddenly becoming constipated or increasing constipation and generalized weakness.

Detection of Cancer of the Rectum and Bowel

Asymptomatic patients can be detected by routine rectal examination, stool for blood tests, and sigmoidoscopy. Early diagnosis is the key to improvement of survival and cure. Routine rectal examination and stool testing for blood must be included in every physical examination, at least on a yearly basis. Ask your doctor to include this as part of the physical. Many times patients themselves discourage the physician from doing this examination, and in these instances the doctor should not be blamed.

Other tests included in the diagnosis of cancer of the bowel and rectum are sigmoidoscopy, barium enema and colonoscopy examinations, and the CEA test.

SIGMOIDOSCOPY

There are few diagnostic examinations which give so much information at a relatively low price as a sigmoidoscopy. The passage of a long, telescopelike tube, called a sigmoidoscope, is uncomfortable but can be life-saving. Many people complain that it is painful and refuse it for that reason. Through this lighted tube one can examine the bowel and see polyps, tumors, and inflammations. Generally it should not take but a few minutes.

Much debate and argument against routine proctosigmoidoscopic examination has come forth for the following reasons: those patients who are below fifty have a relatively low yield of discovered abnormality. Arguments set forth are that massive screening with proctosigmoidoscopy is too expensive, the yield is low, and a stool examination for blood is very sensitive in detecting early cancer. Proctosigmoidoscopy is recommended for high-risk asymptomatic patients who have a positive family history for cancer or known polyps.

THOSE IN FAVOR OF ROUTINE PROCTOSIGMOIDOSCOPY

This is one of the few inexpensive procedures which makes early detection of polyps and cancer possible, thereby increasing the likelihood of their cure. Low yield of positive results is a poor reason when we are dealing with the individual patient.

The essence of medical practice is prevention. Proctosigmoidoscopy need not be performed routinely on someone under forty unless there is a family history of cancer or polyps. Finding polyps in a high percentage of patients forty and over is adequate justification to perform this examination routinely. As mentioned earlier, polyps beyond a certain size are associated with a high incidence of malignancy. It would be shameful if such a simple procedure were abandoned as a routine part of a complete examination. In 100,000 cases of cancer of the rectum and bowel, 50 percent of cancers were detected through a sigmoidoscopy tube.

BARIUM ENEMA

In this X-ray examination of the large intestine a catheter is inserted into the rectum, allowing liquid barium to flow into the rectum and large intestine so pictures can be taken. Prior to the test, patients receive enemas and cathartics to clean the large intestine to assure proper visualization of tumors and inflammation. Patients presenting with rectal bleeding, anemia, or with family history of polyposis need this study, coupled with the proctosigmoidoscope. The sigmoidoscope can visualize areas not clearly seen with the barium enema.

Most internists, surgeons, and cancer specialists look with disfavor on doing routine barium enema examinations as part of executive screening programs.

COLONOSCOPY

This is a study developed by the Japanese that has achieved acceptance during the past ten years. It consists of a long flexible scope, called a *fiberoptic scope,* that is capable of examining the entire colon after its insertion into the rectum. The instrument allows direct inspection of the entire length of the colon in contrast to the proctosigmoidoscope, which only visualizes the first 25 cm. A mass that is identified by barium enema can be readily biopsied in order to study it microscopically and polyps can be removed without having to resort to surgery through the abdomen. Patients with cancer of the rectum or colon who are not completely obstructed should have this examination prior to undergoing surgery, to rule out secondary malignancies which occur in 5 to 10 percent of cases.

The flexible fiberoptic colonoscope has virtually revolutionized diagnostic and therapeutic capabilities in the evaluation of high-risk and symptomatic patients. In patients with premalignant lesions, such as familial polyposis and ulcerative colitis, it has helped to detect early cancer.

Colonoscopy needs to be performed by a physician who is trained and experienced in this procedure.

THE CEA TEST (THE CARCINOEMBRYONIC ANTIGEN)

In some patients bowel cancer produces a substance called CEA, which is an antigen. It is now known that this substance is found in normal serum, normal adult colon tissue, in gastrointestinal malignancies, cirrhosis of the liver, inflammation of the pancreas, and in heavy smokers. It is not a sensitive test for the early detection of cancer, but is useful as a prognostic indicator for cancer of the bowel. The recurrence rate is higher in patients with localized and regional disease who had preoperative CEA levels greater than 5. It seems to be helpful in heralding recurrence of cancer of the colon in the asymptomatic patient, and the test should be performed periodically after surgery.

Treatment of Polyps, Cancer of the Colon and Rectum

Polyps, whether they cause bleeding or not, should be removed. Those in the lower portion of the colon and rectum can be seen and removed through a proctosigmoidoscope. Others in the colon can be removed through the colonoscope. If a malignant polyp is found, some surgeons advise radical treatment: removal of the affected segment of the colon and rectum.

When an abdominal operation for a polyp is suggested, a second opinion is warranted as it is now possible in most cases to remove polyps anywhere in the colon by colonoscopy. If cancer is shown to be invading the base of the polyp, the affected part of the colon should then be removed.

Surgery for Cancer of the Colon and Rectum

The plan of surgery is to remove the tumor mass with enough normal large intestine to ensure that microscopic spread within the wall of the intestine is avoided. If the mass is on the right side of the large intestine, the entire right colon is removed. If it is on the left side, most of the left colon is removed.

Results of Surgery

Cancer involving the inside lining of the colon and not penetrating into the muscular wall has been reported to have a five-year survival rate ranging from 75 to 100 percent. If the tumor penetrates into muscle, the survival rate falls to 60 to 65 percent, and should the tumor extend through all the layers of the large intestine and the surrounding tissue, the survival rate is 40 to 60 percent. If lymph nodes are involved, the five-year survival rate drops to 30 percent. Unfortunately, approximately half of the patients operated on with this common malignancy already have regional lymph node involvement.

Colostomy: Is It Necessary?

Colostomy refers to surgically fixing a portion of the large intestine to the abdominal wall so stool can be collected in a bag. Patients with completely obstructed large intestines may require emergency surgery to construct a colostomy and thereby decompress the large intestine. Occasionally the obstructing tumor mass can be removed at the time that the colostomy is performed. It is generally not good surgical management to attempt to remove the obstructing tumor and then sew the bowel together in the presence of a colon filled with stool. Following the construction of the temporary colostomy, the patient is allowed to recover from surgery and, at a later date, is prepared for elective surgical removal of the tumor.

Cancer of the Rectum

The surgical treatment of cancer of the rectum is an entirely different matter. When the cancer is within 10 cm of the anus, it usually results in removal of the rectum and permanent colostomy. At the present time there are new techniques that allow the surgeon to preserve the rectum and avoid a colostomy using a new stapling device. The stapling device allows the short portion of the rectum to be preserved. It is not known, however, if we are compromising possible cure or long-term survival using this technique. Perhaps in five or ten years the attempt to preserve this short segment of rectum and prevent a colostomy may be abandoned because of a large incidence of recurrent cancer. Surgeons have agonized for years to find a technique to preserve the rectum, as patients' objections to a colostomy are tremendous.

Radiation Therapy

Radiation therapy has been proven to be effective for inoperable or recurrent rectal cancer. Large bulky cancers can be shrunk in size with a four-week course of radiation, as these large masses cannot be removed from the rigid bony structures of the pelvis. Giving preoperative radiation in this situation seems to improve survival rates.

Chemotherapy

The role of chemotherapy in treating colon and rectal cancer that has spread is presently being investigated. Currently there is some indication that chemotherapy may prolong survival time, but only the future will tell.

Follow-Up Care

After an operation with removal of all evidence of cancer of the colon with no evidence of spread beyond the operation site, the patient should be carefully followed. Periodic visits are indicated, including stool testing for blood, along with other blood tests, such as the CEA antigen. Repeated sigmoidoscopy examinations are needed after polyps are removed, as they tend to recur: the removal of the cancer and of the polyps should not end the care of the patient.

DIVERTICULOSIS
AND DIVERTICULITIS

Innocent-looking sacs—which are an out-pouching of the inside lining of the intestinal wall called diverticula—can wreak havoc in the lifetime of a person. An English pathologist called them a "wayside shelter—houses of ill repute where trouble is apt to brew." When these hundreds of little pouches become inflamed, we speak of diverticulitis. Sometimes they form abscesses and other times the blood vessels in these pouches become eroded and there is massive hemorrhage.

Diverticulitis is commonly seen in the later decades of life (fifth through seventh), but diverticulosis becomes evident at a much earlier time, usually is asymptomatic, and found often on a routine barium enema examination.

Mechanism of Formation of Diverticula (Diverticulosis)

This is another medical condition seen primarily in industrialized Western Europe and the United States. It is virtually unknown in underdeveloped countries where the diet is high in vegetables and fruits with little meat—a situation similar to that described for cancer of the colon.

High roughage content causes efficient contraction along the length of the large intestine, called *peristalsis,* which propels the contents through in an orderly fashion, terminating in a normal bowel movement. The cellulose in high vegetable roughage is not digested in man but passes through the intestine as bulk. Remove the bulk of the stool and the muscular action of the intestine becomes disoriented; pressures are exerted against the wall instead of forward. This hypothesis has been confirmed by observing patients who are known to have extensive diverticulosis; if placed on a high roughage diet, they improve, with diminished numbers of diverticula.

Symptoms of Diverticulitis

The patient may have had a long history of constipation or no history of constipation, but for several days complains of crampy abdominal pain, particularly on the left side, sometimes subsiding spontaneously, other times increasing in severity, soon followed by a temperature and chills with nausea and vomiting. The symptoms may be similar to those for appendicitis; diverticulitis has been called appendicitis of the left side. When the pain becomes constant, severe, and localized, an abscess may be present, or a perforation, with a localized inflammation that becomes walled off. The astute physician will suspect diverticulitis in any adult patient with pain in this location and on examination will find tenderness and sometimes a mass in the area of pain. In more severe cases there may even be bowel obstruction.

Medical Management of Diverticulosis and Diverticulitis

Finding asymptomatic diverticulosis in a patient should prompt the physician to encourage the patient to increase the transit time of their bowel movements by having a diet rich in roughage and bulk with the addition of physiological cathartics if they are constipated, to lessen the likelihood of developing diverticulitis. Symptomatic patients with diverticulitis are best managed in a hospital setting.

The usual routine is to give nothing by mouth and administer fluid intravenously with antibiotics until the attack has subsided. To prevent subsequent attacks, patients are again encouraged to follow the African diet of roughage, fruits, bulk, and keeping their bowels open with adequate water intake and physiological cathartics. In more severe cases, if there is an accompanying intestinal obstruction, a tube is passed through the nose that goes into the stomach to decompress the entire intestine and to put it at rest, accompanied by antibiotic treatment until the bowel inflammation subsides.

If an abscess is suggested by the physical findings of a localized swelling or mass, then surgery is advised. Sometimes a cancer may be hiding behind the abscess.

Hemorrhage from Diverticulosis

More often than not, the patient may have been unaware of having diverticulosis and bleed from the rectum. Most of the time bleeding from diverticulosis stops and only requires blood transfusion. Cautious diagnostic procedures are performed at a later date because, again, the preparation for the barium enema, which consists of strong cathartics, can restart the hemorrhage, which may become uncontrollable and force surgery.

The Surgical Point of View

There is little dispute when surgery should be performed, as in cases of local abscess formation, peritonitis, and bowel obstruction that does not improve. The surgeon places a time limit of approximately thirty-six to forty-eight hours on diverticulitis and abscess formation with obstruction. The patient should improve, with fever subsiding, tenderness abating, and the obstruction improving. If not, surgery is performed. Patients with recurrent episodes of diverticulitis closely spaced, causing a great deal of discomfort, annoyance, and repeated hospitalization, fare better by having surgery performed.

The controversy that prevails in this situation is: should surgery be performed for recurrent diverticulitis? Many surgeons recommend surgery once the attack has subsided, with elective resection and removal of the diseased part of the large intestine, after a trial of diligent conservative therapy has failed. Many patients harboring a chronic abscess can only be helped by surgery.

The Type of Surgery Performed

The surgical procedure will depend on the condition of the patient and the presence and extent of abscess formation.

THE THREE-STAGE PROCEDURE

When the abscess is large, with obliteration of the normal anatomy of the left side of the abdomen, it is impossible and dangerous to remove only the abscess. Drainage of the abscess is the best course and with it the stool has to be diverted; otherwise the abscess will never be cleared and the patient will continue to have a contaminated abdomen. To divert the stool, a temporary colostomy is required, and the large intestine above the level of the abscess is brought to the skin of the abdominal wall and opened so the stools can be collected in a bag. These temporary colostomies are set in for six weeks to three months. The colostomy then is closed and the part of the colon that was abscessed is removed.

THE TWO-STAGE PROCEDURE

If the abscess is large but not as bulky as described before, it can be removed along with the segment of the left colon where the infection and diverticula are greatest in number. Approximately 12 to 18 cm are removed and a temporary colostomy is installed. The area is drained and in six weeks to three months a second operation is performed to close the colostomy. This is a more aggressive approach but it does reduce the number of operations to two.

THE ONE-STAGE PROCEDURE

If the pain of diverticulitis continues in spite of excellent treatment in the hospital with bowel rest and intravenous antibiotics, surgery is then performed to remove the area of infection of the left colon and merely sew the two ends of the bowel together. Most of the time this is a rare circumstance and in the authors' experience has occurred only twice in fifteen years.

Summary

At the present time there is little controversy among surgeons and internists about when an operation should be performed. It would be in the interest of the patient to have a medical team of both surgeon and internist, who with back-

and-forth consultations will make the decision as to when an operation is needed. If, after one attack of diverticulitis that subsides, a surgeon recommends resection, a second opinion is warranted.

There is a strong feeling among gastroenterologists, internists, and epidemiologists that diverticulitis could virtually vanish from our Western society if we changed our dietary habits early in childhood. As it is difficult to prescribe such a drastic change without real experimental proof that the condition is indeed caused by decreased roughage in our diet, it would be hard to recommend such a massive program at this time.

15: Cancer of the Lung

IN SPITE OF YEARS OF WARNING about the deadly consequences of cigarette smoking and witnessing great entertainers like John Wayne, Humphrey Bogart, and Walt Disney die of lung cancer, the incidence of cigarette smoking is increasing, and so is cancer of the lung.

When first seen, 50 percent of all patients with this tumor are inoperable and only 5 percent of all lung cancer patients live longer than five years. Now in epidemic proportions, lung cancer was once considered a rarity in earlier times. The disease strikes sixty-four thousand American men and fifteen thousand women. There is irrefutable evidence that one kind of lung cancer, called small cell lung cancer, is related to cigarette smoking. It is almost nonexistent in nonsmokers except those who are exposed to whole body irradiation, uranium miners, and workers exposed to a chemical called chloromethyl ether. Other substances that people work with, such as asbestos, chromium, nickel, iron, isopropyl, and coal tar fumes, increase the risk of cancer. There is extensive research devoted to this illness and the increase of lung cancer continues. Inhaling tobacco smoke from cigarettes remains the most well-known factor.

A man who smokes two packs of cigarettes per day has a one in ten chance of developing cancer of the lung. One study of the residents in New Haven, Connecticut, disclosed a 40 percent greater incidence among the poor than among other economic classes in developing cancer of the lungs. Men living in cities were found to be at greater risk than those who lived in the country. Black men had a higher incidence of lung cancer than white men. A smoker who uses a hookah, like the caterpillar in *Alice's Adventures in Wonderland*, reduces his risk significantly. Recently, low tar cigarettes seem to reduce the incidence of cancer. In the authors' practice, more and more women are found to have lung cancer, a statistic related to dramatically increased cigarette consumption.

The Diagnosis of Cancer of the Lung

These tumors grow silently, more so than any other cancers, and when the first symptoms appear, it is likely that the tumor has spread to other parts of the body. The first symptom described by most patients is an irritating cough occurring at night. Sometimes the first symptom may be seen by a cardiologist when the patient complains of chest pain, later spitting up blood, and shortness of breath, or pneumonia that does not improve.

The majority of lung cancer symptoms come from widespread metastases to bone, liver, and brain. Symptoms may be primarily from these organs. Other times cough, pneumonia, or blood in the sputum may be the first sign.

Traditionally, a chest X ray diagnoses this illness. Once a shadow in the lung is found, other causes must be sought besides cancer, as, for example, tuberculosis. One of the tests included is a sputum examination, in which coughed-up sputum is stained and examined for cancer cells.

Bronchoscopic examination is included as part of the diagnostic workup. This consists of a tube passed through the mouth into the small bronchial tubes. A light at the lower end enables the physician to see the tumor. If he is able to visualize it, he may take a biopsy through the tube. If this fails, the thoracic surgeon inserts a tube into the chest, called a *mediastinoscope*, to search for lymph nodes to biopsy. Seventy-five percent of cases with cancer of the lung will contain cancerous lymph nodes. Other lymph nodes are also biopsied. In particular, the lymph nodes behind the collarbone will be found to contain tumor cells in 25 percent of patients with lung cancer. If the lymph nodes examined show no signs of cancer, there is a cure rate of 40 to 50 percent in patients.

Treatment of Cancer of the Lung

The outlook for this dreaded illness is dismal and the treatment is, on the whole, unsatisfactory. Fewer than 5 percent of patients are cured by any or all methods of treatment.

Chest surgery came into its own in 1930 when good anesthesia was available for open-chest operations, making it possible to operate on lung cancer. Formerly, a radical operation was performed: one lung was removed and as many lymph nodes as possible. Although the surgery was the best for the treatment of the cancer, it was not the best for the survival of the patient. It then became clear that patients do just as well, if not better, if only the affected lobe of the lung is removed, called *lobectomy*. After much bitter debate Dr. R. H. Overholt convinced most surgeons to do only a lobe resection.

The first operation was performed by Dr. Everett Graham in 1933. His patient was a physician who survived twenty-nine years without evidence of cancer. Ironically, Dr. Graham died of lung cancer before the patient.

Present Treatment of Cancer of the Lung

If a lung cancer occupies the central portion, the entire lung is still removed, but if the tumor is at the periphery of the lung, only a small segment of the lung is removed or just the lobe if there is no evidence of spread to lymph nodes. When the surgeon advises removal of the lung in a patient with widespread metastasis, a second opinion should be sought. If the tumor is of the oat cell variety, radiation and chemotherapy may prolong life.

In cancer that has spread far and wide, radiation therapy is now indicated. Radiation therapy is indicated for the relief of symptoms, like coughing up blood, and there is an 80 percent chance of giving the patient some relief. In a small percentage of subjects, if the cancer lesion is not large, it may be completely cured with radiation. In some instances removal of this small tumor by surgery can bring about a cure.

A Look at the Future

At its current rate of increase, it has been estimated that by the year 2000 there will be 300,000 new cases of lung cancer annually. Hope for the future lies in earlier detection of very small tumors by routine chest X ray in high-risk patients, like heavy smokers, combined with sputum analysis. In one study, at New York City Memorial Hospital, 60 percent of patients were cured with early detection of cancer of the lung.

More disheartening surveys recently revealed that in women the incidence of lung cancer is rapidly approaching that of men and may in a few years exceed it. In the authors' own practices the majority of lung cancer cases witnessed in the past two years has been primarily in women who smoke more than one pack of cigarettes per day.

16: Cancer of the Skin

THE AD READ: "Suntanning guaranteed after 20 sessions." Storefront operations with small booths lined with fluorescent sunlamps are appearing all over the country so that we can become a tanned population. Quoting from Gary Trudeau's "Doonesbury" comic strip, the character, Zonker Harris, matched tans with others in the mythical "George Hamilton Cocoa Butter Open." George Hamilton, the actor, was quoted as saying, "It would be a great idea to hold a Cocoa Butter Open."

Suntan is a status symbol of beauty, elegance, and wealth. It is also a future source of a handsome income for the doctor. Of all the cancers in men and women, cancer of the skin is the second most common cancer in the United States. It can kill when untreated. Luckily, dermatologists, surgeons, and oncologists have found ways to cure this widespread malignancy.

If one wants to see the devastating characteristics of this cancer, one should visit the St. Louis Hospital in Paris, which once was a hospital for leprosy and then became the major

European dermatological center. In this hospital, displayed under glass, are models of faces that show the destructive character of skin cancer with its invasion and mutilation of the face, nose, and eyes, penetrating deep into the skull and to the brain. These horror models of historical interest remind us that skin cancer can be devastating if untreated.

The only skin cancer that has a very poor prognosis is the perfidious malignant melanoma, a tumor that develops from a pigmented mole. There is a strong suspicion that President Franklin Delano Roosevelt suffered a malignant melanoma which spread to the right hemisphere of his brain.

Predisposition to Skin Cancer

Lying in the sun is not healthy. The more sun exposure, the more frequent is the incidence of skin cancer. Dangerous sun-ray levels may have increased because of decrease in the ozone layer in our atmosphere.

Certain racial characteristics play a role in determining who develops skin cancer. Men are afflicted more than women, and Scandinavians and North Germans develop this illness more than Arabs, South American Indians, and blacks.

Arsenic exposure in factory workers and in syphilis patients once treated with arsenic compounds leads to cancer of the skin. Tar was the first carcinogenic material identified, found in soot in the eighteenth century. We have seen how chimney sweepers develop various cancers of the lung and rectum; they also develop cancer of the skin and scrotum.

Types of Skin Cancers

There are two major types: squamous cell carcinoma and basal cell carcinoma. The squamous cell has a scaly appearance, slightly raised, with a border that is irregular and may present as a little ulcer. The squamous cell is the one that can sometimes metastasize and grow in other parts of the body.

Basal cell carcinoma, on the other hand, is very similar but it digs into the skin, having the nickname of "rodent ulcer"; it has a central depression with crusting.

The Diagnosis of Skin Cancer

So often either the patient ignores the small abnormality of a skin growth that occurs or sometimes even a doctor may miss it. Some of the most common areas for it to occur are on the face, cheek, or forehead. It is through the biopsy of the lesion that the diagnosis can be made.

Treatment of Cancer of the Skin

Traditionally, surgery and radiation were the only acceptable methods of treatment of skin cancer. Recently, other forms of treatment have become available: the use of local chemicals, electrosurgery (burning), and cryotherapy (freezing).

Dermatologists generally treat skin cancers with electrosurgery and curettage and chemicals. However, chemical treatment has a 50 percent recurrence rate.

It is easy to treat the cancers that occur on the skin of the body or extremities: they are usually simply cut out and the wound is closed. However, if the cancer is very large and occurs on the face or lips, the defect cannot be sutured unless a skin graft is used. Alternative treatments must be made known to the patient, since nonsurgical methods exist. If a surgeon advises wide excision of a cancer of the face with skin graft, a second opinion from a dermatologist is indicated. Chemicals, electrosurgery, and cryotherapy are indicated when the cancer is noninvading.

Surgery is required when the tumor is invading the bone or the cartilage and it is difficult to cure with radiation. If the tumor is present in a conspicuous area, like the lips, the surgeon can remove it, but the lip will obviously not look the same. Radiation in this situation can be just as effective.

17: Tonsillectomy and Adenoidectomy

WE WOULD BE REMISS if we did not include one of the most common operations performed in the United States and probably one of the operations that is most needlessly performed. For fifty years or so, removal of a tonsil was considered a good health measure. Tonsillectomy was also performed for chronic conditions which allegedly are improved by the surgery. Removal of teeth very often accompanied the removal of the tonsils. For example, the treatment of rheumatoid arthritis and osteoarthritis was with tonsillectomy, adenoidectomy, and removal of teeth.

Bad temper, selfishness, ill-behaved children, and slow learners were once treated with tonsillectomy. Pimply children and women who could not conceive or who had too many painful menstrual cramps were advised to have this operation. An attempt by the National Institutes of Health to establish criteria for tonsillectomy recently failed.

Tonsils may become enlarged in early childhood but may not be diseased. As adult life approaches, tonsils tend to undergo a process of involution.

When the adenoids become markedly enlarged, called *hypertrophy*, they may cause the patient to breathe through his open mouth, giving that well-known vacant stupid expression.

The Risk of Tonsillectomy

A number of children still die each year as the result of this operation, and a complication rate as high as 20 percent has been cited, including bleeding and respiratory tract infections.

Indisputable Indications

Indications for performing tonsillectomy are 1) repeated abscess formations in the tissues behind the tonsils, proven by cultures, and 2) tonsils which are so large that they block airways, a condition which is exceedingly rare.

Indications Which Are Not Firm

Conditions which do not necessarily indicate surgery are 1) repeated sore throats in children, even without complications of ear or sinus infections, and 2) incidence of throat infections, inner ear infections, and loss of hearing.

Our opinion is: If the tonsils are markedly enlarged with repeated infections and associated with ear infections and abscess formations, then an operation is indicated. However, streptococcal infections can occur just as frequently after the tonsils are removed. Under no circumstances should tonsils be removed for the treatment of chronic halitosis, rheumatoid arthritis, or thyroid disease.

Indications for Adenoidectomy

The so-called adenoid look described above, resulting from severe obstruction of the nasal passages and recurrent ear infection, is a major indication for removal of adenoids. A second opinion is essential before an operation of tonsillectomy is performed. If a pediatrician suggests it, ask another pediatrician. If a general practitioner suggests it, then ask a pediatrician, and, above all, consult with an ear, nose, and throat specialist before making a final decision.

Snoring is not an indication for the performance of adenoidectomy or tonsillectomy. Most adults do not have adenoid tissues.

18: Hernias of the Groin (Rupture)

NOT ONLY ARE THESE bulbous protrusions unsightly and a favorite subject for comedians, but they can cause serious complications which are not a laughing matter.

A hernia is nothing more than a protrusion of an organ through the wall that normally contains it. When this defect occurs in the groin, it is called an inguinal hernia. The ancient Egyptians in the famed Papyrus Papers describe hernias clearly: ". . . when you judge a swelling on the surface of the body . . . when it comes out . . . caused by coughing." This is not only an affliction of older men but may occur in young men, women, and newborn males.

The surgical correction of inguinal hernias is one of the most commonly performed operations today, exceeded only by hysterectomy. Not all hernias require operations, and a second opinion may be warranted.

Anatomy of a Hernia

As a result of a weakness in the abdominal wall at the groin resulting from disruption or tear of the muscles, the contents of the abdomen slide into a sac, through a canal called the inguinal canal. In the normal individual this canal contains the ducts and tubes connecting to the testicles and to the prostate. The upper portion of this canal may have a weak spot where the abdominal content can travel through and into the groin. The results can be a mere bulge and in others a frank downward slide of the abdominal contents. Other hernias, called abdominal hernias, result from previous surgery and cause a balloonlike swelling at the site of the incision.

Symptoms of a Hernia

The patient may notice a swelling appearing insidiously and increasing in size, generally not associated with any discomfort. Sometimes patients will complain of a nagging ache in the groin. As a rule the abdominal contents slide back and forth and can be easily reduced by pressing the finger into the groin and pushing the contents back upward into the abdomen. As time goes on, the hernia can enlarge and it may not be possible to push it back up, and this is called an incarcerated hernia.

An incarcerated hernia is a true emergency and urgent repair is indicated, as the blood supply can be cut off by the pressure from the ring of the hernia. The bowel or other tissue can then become gangrenous with the escape of bacteria into the bloodstream, causing a life-threatening generalized infection. In this situation the patient may complain of severe pain which may at first have been intermittent but then becomes persistent.

Precipitating Causes for Hernias to Form

Improper lifting of heavy objects from a bent position can cause a hernia if there is a weakness of the sac. Heavy smokers with chronic coughs and patients with severe chronic pulmonary disease have a tendency to form hernias. Sometimes the appearance of the hernia may signal the presence of a cancer of the bowel. It is imperative that the patient query his physician regarding the possibility of an underlying malignancy.

The Treatment of Inguinal Hernias:
The Surgical Point Of View

For centuries, because the anatomy was not thoroughly known, correction could rarely be achieved successfully and patients invariably resorted to trusses. Surgical intervention was considered so dangerous that it was rarely attempted, until the famous American surgeon, William Halsted, devised the first successful operation in the late 1800s. (Halsted was mentioned earlier as being credited with performing the first radical mastectomy.)

Halsted was a very unusual man. Trained at Yale and Johns Hopkins, he became a legendary figure in surgery, and performed many heroic acts. In 1881, when his sister was hemorrhaging, Halsted withdrew blood from his own vein and injected it into her. When his mother was critically ill with gallbladder disease and no other surgeon would operate, Halsted saved her life by removing multiple gallstones, although he had never before operated on a gallbladder.

Unfortunately, Halsted, besides performing the first successful hernia operation in 1889, became interested in the use of cocaine as a local anesthetic. To test its efficacy, he began to inject it into himself. Then he switched to morphine and his addiction ruined his life. His gregarious and gay manners changed and he became a sullen, depressed surgeon. He continued to operate vigorously, making brilliant innovations, but it was never known for certain if he overcame his addiction. He died from a complication of gallbladder surgery in 1922.

Most surgeons feel that hernias should be repaired to avoid the devastating consequences of incarceration and strangulation, which can make the operation exceedingly risky and lead to death.

Choice of Anesthesia

Traditionally, hernia operations were performed with general anesthesia, but today most hernias can be repaired under local anesthesia with the patient mildly sedated. This is not done routinely for two reasons: the surgeon may be uncomfortable using local anesthesia for such a major procedure, which lasts from forty-five minutes to one and a half hours, or the patient would rather not witness the ordeal. Some surgeons insist that all hernia repairs be done under local anesthesia. The final choice should be with the patient. Obese patients and those with recurrent hernias fare better with general or spinal anesthesia.

The Shouldice Clinic in Toronto has received a great deal of publicity in the treatment of hernias. Their technique has received moderate acceptance in the United States. The procedure is short and there is a very brief period of convalescence. At this clinic an extensive training program is carried out for the patient preoperatively and postoperatively for early ambulation and minimal use of medication for pain.

The Medical Point of View

We fully agree that large bulging hernias should be operated on to avoid the complication of incarceration and strangulation. Small bulges can be watched and may never need surgery. Abdominal hernias, as a rule, are left alone, except for cosmetic reasons.

Patients suffering from prostatic problems who have to exert force to urinate can also cause the appearance of a hernia, as can patients with chronic cough. If these conditions are not alleviated or corrected, there may be a recurrence of the hernia.

Individuals who have had hernias all their lives and are suffering from heart, lung, or kidney disease, or other major illnesses, should seek a second opinion before having surgery. Some older patients have worn a truss for a long time and have fared well with it and should not be advised to have surgery.

Finally, we favor local anesthesia whenever it is possible.

Recurrence of Hernia

The incidence of recurrent inguinal hernia is difficult to know. As a rule, surgeons say they rarely see a recurrent hernia in their own patients. The patient, in fact, may not return to the same surgeon, for he feels that the surgeon has failed and will therefore go to another surgeon for a second repair.

Estimated recurrence rates have been calculated to be approximately 5 to 10 percent. Recurrence of hernia can be avoided if proper care is taken postoperatively. The patient must allow six to eight weeks of limited activity to assure strong wound healing. During the convalescent period walking is acceptable but lifting or repetitive working, such as painting or vacuuming, is discouraged. Once there is recurrence, the incidence increases with each repair.